Ketogenic Diet:

150+ Low-Carb, Rapid Fat Loss Keto Recipes & Desserts You Can Try At Home! (Burn Fat, Lose Weight, Ketogenic Recipes, Ketogenic Cookbook, Ketogenic Fat Bombs)

Kevin Moore © 2017

Introduction

First off, thanks for purchasing my book "Ketogenic Diet: 150+ Low-Carb, Rapid Fat Loss Keto Recipes & Desserts You Can Try At Home!" By deciding to pick up this book it shows that you're ready to make living a healthier lifestyle a priority going forward. This book will provide you with a ton of healthy and delicious ketogenic recipes. I hope this keto diet has the same type of positive impact on your life that it had on mine. I lost a bunch of weight while also getting my blood pressure and blood sugar under control. Today, I start each morning with more energy and I'm able to lead a fuller life because of the recipes I'm about to share with you.

It's always important before beginning any new diet that you talk to your physician. The ketogenic diet isn't meant for everyone. I'm not a doctor, I'm just a guy who's had a moderate amount of success with the ketogenic diet. I've found that it allowed me to quickly and safely lose weight while also helping get my other health issues under better control. I hope you enjoy the variety of recipes I've included in this guide. They should keep you eating healthy for the foreseeable future.

I'm excited to get started. Let's begin!

Chapter One: Ketogenic Diet Breakfast Recipes

In this section, I will give you 30+ keto breakfast recipes you can make yourself. I'll include both basic recipes and a few more advanced recipes. That way no matter what your level is in the kitchen you'll be able to prepare yourself a healthy low-carb ketogenic meal to keep you on track with your diet. I'll add in the nutritional value whenever possible, although I don't always have those exact numbers for each and every recipe.

Breakfast Keto Pizza (Serves 2)

Ingredients:

10 slices of Pepperoni

4 Eggs

2 ounces of Cheddar Cheese

4 slices of Bacon

Onion Powder

Garlic Powder

Pepper

Salt

Directions:

1. Cook your bacon and reserve your bacon grease in your skillet.

2. Let your pan cool off for a bit.

3. Crack your eggs into your pan and put them all close together.

4. Apply your seasoning.

5. Cook at 450 degrees in your oven for approximately 6 minutes. Add your toppings and cheddar.

6. Cook for approximately 4 more minutes. Place your bacon on top.

7. Serve!

Nutritional Value:

307 Calories.

22 grams of Protein.

1 gram of Carbs.

24 grams of Fat.

Breakfast Meatloaf (Serves 4)

Ingredients:

6 Large Eggs

4 ounces of Organic Cream Cheese (Room Temperature)

1 pound of Sweet Italian Sausage or Breakfast Sausage

1 cup of Shredded Cheddar Cheese

1/4 Yellow Onion (Chopped)

2 tablespoons of Chopped Scallion

Ghee

Directions:

1. Preheat your oven to 350 degrees.

2. Grease your small-sized loaf pan with your ghee.

3. In your large-sized bowl, lightly beat your eggs. Add your sausage, onion, and half of your cream cheese. Mix together thoroughly.

4. Pour your meatloaf and egg mixture into your loaf pan. Add to your oven and bake, uncovered, for approximately 30 minutes or until stiff.

5. Remove from your oven and allow it to sit for about 5 minutes. Some of your fat may have risen up to the top and begun to cool. You can use your spoon to lightly scrape it off.

6. Spread your remaining cream cheese over the top of your meatloaf, then top it with your scallions and cheddar cheese. Add your meatloaf back to the oven.

7. Bake for approximately 5 minutes, then switch to broil for about 2 to 3 minutes or until your cheddar cheese begins to golden and crisp.

8. Remove from your oven. Allow your meatloaf to rest for at least 5 minutes before slicing.

9. Serve!

Nutritional Value:

682 Calories.

38 grams of Protein.

5 grams of Carbs.

56 grams of Fat.

Keto Cinnamon Crunchy Granola (Serves 4)

Ingredients:

1 cup of Sliced Almonds

1 cup of Diced Walnuts

1 cup of Unsweetened Coconut Flakes

2 tablespoons of Melted Coconut Oil

4 packs of Splenda Naturals

2 teaspoons of Cinnamon

Directions:

1. Preheat your oven to 375 degrees.

2. Line your baking sheet with your parchment paper.

3. In your medium-sized bowl, toss all your ingredients together.

4. Spread out your mixture over your baking sheet in as close to a single layer as you can.

5. Add to your oven and bake for approximately 10 minutes, or until your mixture begins to brown.

6. Remove, mix again and place in your bowl with some cold unsweetened almond milk.

7. Serve!

Nutritional Value:

562 Calories.

14 grams of Protein.

16 grams of Carbs.

54 grams of Fat.

Keto Cacao Nibs Cereal (Serves 4)

Ingredients:

2 tablespoons of Raw Cacao Nibs

1/2 cup of Chia Seeds

4 tablespoons of Hemp Hearts

2 tablespoons of Melted Coconut Oil

1 tablespoon of Fine Psyllium Powder

1 tablespoon of Organic Vanilla Extract

1 cup of Water

1 tablespoon of Swerve

Directions:

1. Preheat your oven to 285 degrees.

2. In your large-sized mixing bowl, combine your chia seeds and water, stir well and allow it to sit for approximately 5 minutes.

3. Add the rest of your ingredients to your bowl, except for the cacao nibs.

4. With your electric mixer or wooden spoon, mix all your ingredients together well until they are evenly amalgamated.

5. Add your cacao nibs and stir them into your dough. The dough should form a nice ball of pliable consistency.

6. Roll out 2 large-sized pieces of oven paper, about 11x14-inches.

7. Take your dough and using your hands form it into a cylinder. Place it on your parchment paper with the shiny side up.

8. With your fingers start flattening the dough. Cover it with the other piece of your paper, shiny side down, and roll it out with a rolling pin to a thickness of 1/4 to 1/8-inch.

9. Gently peel off the top paper from your dough. Lay your dough on top of the paper on your cookie sheet or the top part of your broiler pan.

10. Bake on one side for approximately 15 minutes or until almost dry. Remove from your oven and carefully flip your sheet of dough. It should be dry enough to remove your oven paper, peeling it gently.

11. Bake for another 15 to 25 minutes or until dry. Remove from your oven and allow it to cool.

12. Using a large kitchen knife cut your cereal into 1-inch squares.

13. Serve!

Nutritional Value:

254 Calories.

9 grams of Protein.

1.5 grams of Carbs.

15.5 grams of Fat.

Keto Scrambled Eggs (Serves 2)

Ingredients:

6 Eggs

4 strips of Bacon

2 tablespoons of Sour Cream

1/2 teaspoon of Onion Powder

1/2 teaspoon of Garlic Powder

2 tablespoons of Butter

1/4 teaspoon of Paprika

1/4 teaspoon of Black Pepper

1/2 teaspoon of Salt

Green Onion (Optional)

Directions:

1. Crack your eggs into your ungreased, cold pan and then add your butter. Wait to mix your eggs until you put the heat on. Don't season your eggs until after they are cooked. It will break them down and make them watery instead of creamy.

2. Put your pan on a medium-high heat. Start stirring your butter and eggs together using your silicone spatula. While stirring your eggs, cook some bacon strips in a different pan to your desired level of crispiness.

3. Alternate stirring your eggs both on heat and off the heat. A few seconds on and a few seconds off the flame. If the eggs begin cooking in a thin, dry looking layer at the bottom of your pan, take if off heat. Scrape it using your spatula and that thin layer should regain some of its creaminess.

4. Once your eggs are almost done turn off the flame. Your eggs will still cook a little more due to the residual heat in your pan.

5. Add 2 tablespoons of your sour cream. Season your eggs using your pepper, salt, garlic powder, paprika, and onion powder.

6. Add in a couple stalks of chopped green onion for some contrasting flavor if you so desire.

7. Serve!

Nutritional Value:

444 Calories.

25 grams of Protein.

2 grams of Carbs.

35 grams of Fat.

Deep Fried Eggs (Serves 1)

Ingredients:

3 slices of Bacon

2 Eggs

Directions:

1. Heat your oil in your deep fryer to approximately 375 degrees.

2. Cook your bacon.

3. Crack your eggs into your prep bowl.

4. Slip your egg into the center of your fryer. Don't drop eggs in, try to slip your eggs in near the surface.

5. Using 2 different spatulas, corral your eggs into a ball. This may take a little practice to get the hang of.

6. Fry for approximately 3 to 4 minutes or until the bubbling stops.

7. Drain on your paper towels.

8. Serve!

Nutritional Value:

321 Calories.

27 grams of Protein.

1 gram of Carbs.

24 grams of Fat.

One Skillet Eggs & Bacon

Ingredients:

4 Large Eggs

1/2 cup of Shredded Colby Jack Cheese

8 slices of Bacon

1/2 cup of Chopped Cauliflower or Broccoli

1 tablespoon of Butter

1/2 cup of Finely Chopped Celery

1/2 Large Chopped White Onion.

1 Peeled Carrot

Directions:

1. Slice your bacon across its grain into smaller-sized strips.

2. Melt your butter in your large-sized skillet over a medium heat.

3. Add your bacon and vegetables.

4. Stir often and saute your vegetables and bacon in your butter for approximately 20 minutes. You want your bacon to begin crisping on its edges and you want your vegetables to being caramelizing.

5. Spread your mixture over your skillet as evenly as possible and make 4 wells one in each quarter of your skillet.

6. Break an egg into each of the wells. Cook your eggs until they are nearly done. Cook shorter if you like your yolks runny and longer if you like them harder.

7. When your eggs are nearly done sprinkle cheese on top and allow it to cook until your cheese melts and the eggs are done.

8. Serve!

Ricotta Scrambled Eggs (Serves 1)

Ingredients:

2 Eggs

2 ounces of Italian Dry Salami

5 ounces of 2% Fat Ricotta Cheese

1 tablespoon of Olive Oil

1 teaspoon of Rosemary

Salt

Pepper

Directions:

1. Chop your salami up into smaller-sized cubes. Fry them together in your small-sized pan using olive oil.

2. While frying, whisk your eggs, add your salt, pepper, and rosemary.

3. Add your ricotta into your egg mixture, mix together well to break up any large-sized lumps.

4. Add your eggs and ricotta mixture to your pan and cook for approximately 5 minutes until done.

5. Serve!

Nutritional Value:

598 Calories.

28 grams of Protein.

5 grams of Carbs.

45 grams of Fat.

Keto Sausage & Egg Muffin (Serves 1)

Ingredients:

Muffin:

1 Egg

1 tablespoon Coconut Flour

1 tablespoon Almond Milk

1/2 teaspoon Baking Powder

1/2 tablespoon Olive Oil

1 pinch of Salt

Filling:

1 Sausage Link

1 slice of Cheese

1 Egg

1/4 teaspoon of Sage

1/4 teaspoon of Thyme

1/8 teaspoon of Black Pepper

1/4 teaspoon of Salt

Directions:

1. Preheat your oven to 400 degrees.

2. Crack your egg into your mixing bowl and add each of your muffin ingredients.

3. Mix together well. Get rid of any clumps and pour your batter into your ramekin. Bake for approximately 15 minutes.

4. Crack your egg into your ramekin. Give your egg a good stir and season with your salt and pepper. Bake for approximately 10 minutes.

5. Cut open your pork sausage link and discard its casing.

6. Add your seasonings to your sausage meat and mix using your hands. Shape them into a patty and then cook using your hot pan for approximately 4 to 5 minutes on both sides.

7. Remove from the oven and cut your muffins into thin halves. Toast them until they are browned.

8. Put together your sandwich and add your slice of cheese.

9. Serve!

Nutritional Value:

460 Calories.

29 grams of Protein.

3 grams of Carbs.

37 grams of Fat.

Cali Chicken Omelet (Serves 1)

Ingredients:

1 ounce of Deli Cut Chicken

2 Eggs

1 Campari Tomato

2 slices of Bacon (Chopped & Cooked)

1 tablespoon of Mayo

1/4 Avocado

1 teaspoon of Mustard

Directions:

1. Crack your eggs and beat them in your small-sized bowl. Add to your hot pan. Pull sides of your eggs towards the center to cook your omelet faster. Season them with your pepper and salt.

2. Once your eggs are half cooked, should take approximately 5 minutes, add your bacon, tomato, chicken, and sliced avocado. Add in your mayo and mustard.

3. Fold your omelet over onto itself. Cover using your lid. Cook until finished. Should take approximately 5 minutes.

4. Serve!

Nutritional Value:

415 Calories.

25 grams of Protein.

4 grams of Carbs.

32 grams of Fat.

Breakfast Lettuce Taco (Serves 2)

Ingredients:

4 Large Eggs

6 slices of Bacon

2 slices of Cheddar Cheese

2 tablespoons of Heavy Cream

2 tablespoons of Shredded Cheddar

2 Romaine Lettuce Leafs

Onion Powder

Pepper

Salt

Directions:

1. Cook your bacon to your desired preference.

2. Whisk your eggs, cream, and add your seasonings.

3. Scramble your eggs and mix in your cheese at the end.

4. Combine your eggs, cheese, bacon, and lettuce.

5. Serve!

Nutritional Value:

499 Calories.

29 grams of Protein.

3 grams of Carbs.

40 grams of Fat.

Iced Matcha Latte (Serves 1)

Ingredients:

1 teaspoon of Matcha Powder

1 tablespoon of Coconut Oil

1/8 teaspoon of Vanilla Bean

1 cup of Unsweetened Cashew Milk

2 Ice Cubes

Directions:

1. Combine all of your ingredients in your blender and continue to blend until your ice cubes are broken up.

2. Sprinkle some extra matcha on top as a garnish.

3. Serve!

Nutritional Value:

148 Calories.

1 gram of Protein.

0.5 grams of Carbs.

15 grams of Fat.

Keto Hemp Heart Porridge (Serves 1)

Ingredients:

1 cup of Non-Dairy Milk

2 tablespoons of Freshly Ground Flax Seed

1/2 cup of Manitoba Harvest Hemp Hearts

1 tablespoon of Xylitol

1 tablespoon of Chia Seeds

3/4 teaspoon of Pure Vanilla Extract

1/4 cup of Crushed Almonds or Almond Flour

1/2 teaspoon of Ground Cinnamon

Toppings:

1 tablespoon of Manitoba Harvest Hemp Hearts

3 Brazil Nuts

Directions:

1. Add all of your ingredients but your almonds and toppings to your small-sized saucepan. Stir well until combined, then heat over a medium heat until it begins to lightly boil. No need to cover.

2. Once lightly bubbling, stir once over and leave it to cook for another 1 to 2 minutes.

3. Remove from the heat, stir in your crushed almonds and drop into your bowl. Top with your toppings.

4. Serve!

Feta & Pesto Omelet (Serves 1)

Ingredients:

3 Eggs

1 ounce of Feta Cheese

1 tablespoon of Butter

1 tablespoon of Pesto

1 tablespoon of Heavy Cream

Salt

Pepper

Directions:

1. Melt a tablespoon of your butter in your pan and allow it to heat up.

2. Beat your eggs in your bowl with a tablespoon of heavy cream.

3. Pour your eggs into your hot pan and cook until nearly done.

4. Sprinkle your feta cheese on half of the omelet. Spread a tablespoon of pesto on the same half.

5. Fold your omelet over onto itself. Cook for approximately 4 to 5 minutes so that your feta cheese all melts and your eggs cook properly.

6. Garnish with more feta cheese on top.

7. Serve!

Nutritional Value:

570 Calories.

30 grams of Protein.

2.5 grams of Carbs.

46 gram of Fat.

Spinach Egg White Omelet

Ingredients:

5 Egg Whites

1 Plum Tomato

1 Egg Yolk

2 tablespoons of Almond Milk

1 tablespoon of Purple Onion

Pinch of Basil

Handful of Shredded Spinach

Olive Oil Cook Spray

Garlic (Optional)

Directions:

1. Chop up your vegetables.

2. Beat your egg whites, yolk, and almond milk.

3. Spray your small-sized frying pan with your olive oil spray and saute your vegetables until they get soft.

4. Put your vegetables to the side.

5. Spray your pan again with olive oil spray.

6. Place the heat on a medium-low and pour in your egg mixture. Cook your eggs until firm, then add your vegetables on one side of eggs and fold the other side of your eggs over top.

7. Add to your plate.

8. Serve!

Nutritional Value:

203 Calories.

20 grams of Protein.

18 grams of Carbs.

5 grams of Fat.

Spicy Shrimp Omelet (Serves 2)

Ingredients:

10 Large Shrimp

6 Eggs

4 Grape Tomatoes

1/4 Onion

1 tablespoon of Sriracha Salt

1 teaspoon of Cayenne

Handful of Spinach

Sprig of Parsley

Directions:

1. Chop your onion and slice your grape tomatoes lengthwise in half.

2. Fire your pan to a medium heat. Add your onions and salt. Add your grape tomatoes cut side down so they can roast a little bit.

3. When your onions get translucent add in your spinach and allow it to shrink and wilt enough for some of your shrimp to fit in.

4. Throw your shrimp in.

5. Crack each egg leaving room for all of them. Take your spoon and jiggle around the whites so they grab everything that is underneath them.

6. Place a lid on your pan. Allow your omelet to cook for approximately 6 to 8 minutes. Watch your eggs, once thin film of white has covered the yolks they're ready. If your eggs are still runny allow them to cook a bit longer.

7. Once your omelet is done, run your knife across each of the yolks and allow them to ooze out onto your whole omelet. Garnish with your parsley.

8. Serve!

<u>Nutritional Value:</u>

329 Calories.

36 grams of Protein.

4 grams of Carbs.

17 grams of Fat.

Cast Iron Skillet Frittata (Serves 8)

Ingredients:

12 Eggs

8 slices of Bacon

1 Small Pepper

12 ounces of Cheddar Cheese

1 Small Onion

6 ounces of Heavy Cream

1/2 teaspoon of Onion Powder

19 ounces of Brussels Sprouts

1/2 teaspoon of Garlic Powder

1 head of Cauliflower

1/2 teaspoon of Salt

1/2 teaspoon of Pepper

Directions:

1. Cook your bacon until it's crisp. Keep your bacon grease in your skillet.

2. Thinly slice your pepper and onion.

3. Shred your cauliflower and brussels sprouts.

4. Cook your vegetables in your skillet.

5. While your veggies are cooking, prepare your egg mixture with eggs, spices, and cream. Whisk them together to combine.

6. When your vegetables are finished they should be translucent and cooked. Crumble and add in your cheese and bacon.

7. Mix together and add in your eggs. Mix it again.

8. Cook approximately 2 to 3 minutes on your stove top.

9. Transfer over to your skillet and cook in your oven for approximately 25 minutes at 450 degrees.

10. Take out of your oven and slice.

11. Serve!

Nutritional Value:

491 Calories.

29 grams of Protein.

18 grams of Carbs.

35 grams of Fat.

Strawberry Almond Milk (Serves 2)

Ingredients:

16 ounces of Unsweetened Almond Milk

1/4 cup of Unsweetened Frozen Strawberries

4 ounces of Heavy Cream

1 scoop of Whey Vanilla Isolate Powder

Stevia or Low-Carb Sweetener

Directions:

1. Put each of your ingredients in your blender.

2. Blend together until it is smooth.

3. Serve!

Nutritional Value:

304 Calories.

15 grams of Protein.

7 grams of Carbs.

25 grams of Fat.

High Fiber Coffee & Coconut Cup (Serves 1)

Ingredients:

1 ounce of Unsweetened Ground Flaxseed

1 ounce of Ground Flaxseed

1/2 cup of Unsweetened Black Coffee

1 tablespoon of Coconut Oil

Liquid Sweetener

Directions:

1. Mix your flaxseed and coconut flakes together well.

2. Add your coconut oil. Pour your hot coffee on it and mix. Adjust the level of thickness by adding more still water or coffee.

3. Add 3 to 4 drops of liquid sweetener.

4. Serve!

Nutritional Value:

277 Calories.

4 grams of Protein.

7 grams of Carbs.

27 grams of Fat.

Fried Crusty Cheddar (Serves 1)

Ingredients:

1 Egg

1 teaspoon of Ground Flaxseed

2 slices of Cheddar Cheese

1 teaspoon of Almond Flour

1 tablespoon of Olive Oil

1 teaspoon of Hemp Nuts

Salt

Pepper

Directions:

1. Heat your olive oil in your frying pan over a medium heat.

2. Whisk your egg with your pepper and salt.

3. Mix your flaxseed with your hemp nuts and almond flour.

4. Coat your cheddar slices with your egg mixture and then with your dry mixture.

5. Fry them for approximately 3 minutes on both sides.

6. Serve!

<u>Nutritional Value:</u>

588 Calories.

35 grams of Protein.

5 grams of Carbs.

48 grams of Fat.

Cajun Hash (Serves 2)

Ingredients:

8 ounces of Shaved Red Pastrami (Chopped Into 1-Inch Slices)

1/2 Onion

1 Egg

1 pound bag of Frozen Cauliflower (Chopped Into Even Small-Sized Chunks)

2 tablespoons of Minced Garlic

1/2 Green Pepper (Chopped Into 1/4-Inch Slices)

1 teaspoon of Cajun Seasoning

2 tablespoons of Ghee or Olive Oil

Directions:

1. In your ghee or olive oil, saute your chopped onions for approximately 5 minutes on a medium heat.

2. After 5 minutes, saute your garlic for approximately 2 minutes.

3. Squeeze out any excess water from your chopped cauliflower. Add it to your saute and cook for approximately 5 to 10 minutes. It will be done once it's crispy and brown.

4. Add your Cajun seasoning and mix in.

5. Add your green peppers and your chopped pastrami.

6. Toss and cook until it's hot all around. Should take approximately 5 minutes. Add to your bowl.

7. Fry your egg sunny side up. Add to the top of your hash. Dash with your Cajun seasoning.

8. Serve!

Onion & Cheese Quiche (Serves 12)

Ingredients:

12 Large Organic Eggs

1 Large White Onion (Finely Chopped)

6 cups of Shredded Colby Jack Cheese or Muenster Cheese

2 tablespoons of Butter

2 teaspoons of Dried Thyme

2 cups of Heavy Cream

1 teaspoon of Ground Black Pepper

1 teaspoon of Salt

Directions:

1. Prepare your oven to 350 degrees.

2. In your large-sized skillet add your butter and melt over a medium-low heat.

3. Add your vegetables and saute until your onions are soft and translucent.

4. Remove them from your heat and allow it to cool.

5. Butter 2 of your deep pie pans or 10-inch quiche pans. Put in 2 cups of your shredded cheese to cover the bottom of each of your buttered pans.

6. Add 1/2 of your cooled vegetable mixture to each one of your pans. Make sure they are evenly layered over your cheese.

7. Crack all of your eggs and pour them into your large-sized mixing bowl.

8. Add your spices and cream together. Whisk until frothy and well mixed.

9. Pour 1/2 of your mixture over each pan and use your fork to evenly distribute the cheese and veggies into your egg and cream mix.

10. Slide your pans into your oven. Leave about an inch between your pans. Continue to bake for approximately 20 to 25 minutes. Should be slightly golden colored in the middle and puffy looking.

11. Remove from your oven and cut each of your quiches into 6 servings of equal size. Can last to up to a week when refrigerated.

12. Serve!

Nutritional Value:

382 Calories.

16 grams of Protein.

4 grams of Carbs.

33 grams of Fat.

Clouds of Eggs (Serves 4)

Ingredients:

4 Large Eggs

2 tablespoons of Parmesan Cheese

2 slices of Bacon

Garlic Powder

Onion Powder

Salt

Pepper

Directions:

1. Split your egg yolks from your egg whites.

2. Cut up your bacon and cook for some bacon bits.

3. Put your eggs in your bowl and then whip them until they are stiff.

4. Shred your Parmesan cheese into your egg whites and then add in your bacon bits.

5. Split your egg white into 4 separate mounds on your parchment paper or a silicon mat.

6. Bake your egg whites for approximately 5 minutes at 350 degrees until they are set.

7. Put your egg yolk into each of your mounds.

8. Bake your egg whites until brown.

9. Serve!

Nutritional Value:

98 Calories.

6 grams of Protein.

1 gram of Carbs.

7 grams of Fat.

Ricotta Cheese w/ Vanilla (Serves 1)

Ingredients:

7 ounces of 2% Fat Ricotta Cheese

1 tablespoon of Creme Fraiche

1 sachet of Vanilla Flavoring

Directions:

1. Mix your ricotta with your creme fraiche and vanilla flavoring.

2. Serve!

Nutritional Value:

290 Calories.

8 grams of Protein.

3 grams of Carbs.

18 grams of Fat.

Breakfast Chorizo Casserole (Serves 10)

Ingredients:

12 Eggs

8 ounces of Cheddar

1 Small Onion

16 ounces of Ground Chorizo

12 tablespoons of Heavy Cream

13 ounces of Spinach

1 Small Pepper

1 teaspoon of Garlic Powder

9 ounces of Cherry Tomatoes

1 teaspoon of Onion Powder

1 teaspoon of Salt

1 teaspoon of Pepper

Directions:

1. Cook your spinach in your microwave.

2. Chop or grind up your chorizo and then cook it in your skillet until it is browned.

3. Place your finished chorizo in your large-sized bowl.

4. Thinly slice your pepper and onion. Cook them in the same skillet. Place in your large-sized bowl when finished.

5. Add your finished spinach to your bowl.

6. Whisk together your eggs, spices, and heavy cream.

7. Add your cheese to your bowl and then combine. Add your egg mixture.

8. Transfer to your greased casserole dish.

9. Add your cherry tomatoes.

10. Cook for approximately 50 minutes at 350 degrees. Remove from your oven.

11. Serve!

Nutritional Value:

362 Calories.

24 grams of Protein.

7 grams of Carbs.

28 grams of Fat.

Steak & Eggs (Serves 1)

Ingredients:

4 ounces of Sirloin

3 Eggs

1/4 Avocado

1 tablespoon of Butter

Salt

Pepper

Directions:

1. Melt your butter in your pan. Fry your eggs until the whites have been set and the yolk is done to your desired preference. Season them with your pepper and salt.

2. Cook your sirloin in another pan until done to your desired preference. Slice into small-sized strips and season with your pepper and salt.

3. Slice up your avocado and add to your dish.

4. Serve!

<u>Nutritional Value:</u>

510 Calories.

44 grams of Protein.

3 grams of Net Carbs.

26 grams of Fat.

Sour Cream Blueberry Muffins (Serves 15)

Ingredients:

2 Eggs

1 cup of Sour Cream

2 cups of Almond Flour

4 ounces of Fresh Blueberries

1/4 cup of Erythritol

1/8 cup of Melted Butter

1/2 teaspoon of Baking Soda

1/2 teaspoon of Salt

Directions

1. Preheat your oven to 350 degrees. Put your cupcake papers in each muffin hole of your 12 count muffin pan. You'll want to use 2 of these pans as your recipe will produce 15 muffins.

2. Whisk your dry ingredients and almond flour together.

3. In a different bowl, lightly beat your eggs and then mix in your butter and sour cream until smooth.

4. Add your almond flour mix and sour cream mix together and stir well.

5. Add in your blueberries and stir until they are distributed evenly.

6. Spoon your mixture in each of your muffin cups. Fill them 1/2 full.

7. Bake for approximately 20 minutes. They are considered done once they turn a golden color.

8. Allow them to cool off.

9. Serve!

<u>Nutritional Value:</u>

147 Calories.

5 grams of Protein.

5 grams of Carbs.

13 grams of Fat.

Two Cheese Muffins (Serves 15)

Ingredients:

2 Eggs

1/2 cup of Shredded Muenster

2 cups of Almond Flour

1/2 cup of Shredded Muenster

1/2 teaspoon of Baking Soda

1 cup of Sour Cream

1/2 teaspoon of Dried Thyme

1 cup of Shredded Cheddar

1/8 cup of Melted Butter

1/4 teaspoon of Salt

Directions:

1. Preheat your oven to 400 degrees. Place your cupcake papers in each muffin hole on your normal size 12 count muffin pan.

2. Whisk your dry ingredients and almond flour together.

3. In a different bowl, lightly beat your eggs and mix in your butter and sour cream.

4. Add your liquid mixture to your almond flour mix. If your batter seems a little too thick add a tablespoon of heavy cream or water.

5. Add your cheese and stir until it is distributed evenly.

6. Spoon your mixture into your muffin cups. Each should be filled 3/4 of the way.

7. Bake for approximately 5 minutes at 400 degrees.

8. Turn down your oven temperature to 350 degrees and bake it for another 20 minutes or until it is golden.

9. Take it out of your oven and allow it to cool down.

10. Serve!

Nutritional Value:

166 Calories.

6 grams of Protein.

5 grams of Carbs.

15 grams of Fat.

Delightful Scrambled Eggs

Ingredients:

3 Large Eggs

1 tablespoon of Unsalted Butter

Coarse Salt

Fresh Ground Pepper

Directions:

1. Beat your eggs using your fork.

2. Melt your butter using a nonstick medium skillet over a low heat.

3. Add in your egg mixture.

4. Using your spatula (preferably flexible and heatproof), gently move your eggs into the center of your pan and allow the liquid parts to run out to the perimeter. Continue to cook moving your eggs with your spatula until they are set. Should take approximately 1 1/2 minutes to 3 minutes.

5. Season your eggs with your pepper and salt.

6. Serve!

Nutritional Value:

318 Calories.

17.5 grams of Protein.

1.8 grams of Carbs.

26.3 grams of Fat.

Keto Bacon Pancakes (Serves 8)

Ingredients:

1 Egg

1/2 cup of Heavy Cream

8 slices of Bacon

1/4 cup of Water

1 tablespoon of Sugar-Free Vanilla Syrup

1/2 cup of Melted Unsalted Butter

1 cup of Carbquik

1/2 teaspoon of Baking Soda

Directions:

1. Cook your bacon.

2. Melt your butter in your microwave.

3. Mix together your baking soda and Carbquik.

4. Add your liquid ingredients and mix it all together.

5. Heat your pan over a medium-high heat. Spray it with Pam.

6. Spoon some batter into your pan. Don't make the pancake so large you can't flip it. Add your bacon.

7. When your edges brown or bubbles form in the center flip your pancake.

8. Continue to cook for another minute until the center is cooked. Check with your fork.

9. Remove your pancakes and make the next one.

10. Repeat the process until all your pancakes are finished.

11. Serve!

Nutritional Value:

443 Calories.

12 grams of Protein.

5 grams of Carbs.

46 grams of Fat.

Raspberry Protein Pancakes

Ingredients:

1/4 cup of Egg Whites

1 scoop of Whey Protein Powder

1/2 Banana

1 tablespoon of Cinnamon

2 tablespoons of Almond Milk

2 tablespoons of Greek Yogurt

3/4 cup of Raspberries

1 tablespoon of Chia Seeds

Directions:

1. Mash up your banana.

2. Grind up your chia seeds.

3. Add all your ingredients except your raspberries to your bowl and stir together well.

4. Add your raspberries and stir.

5. Spray your small-sized pan with some olive oil spray and then pour in your mix.

6. Cook your pancakes on a medium heat until your edges are brown. Once this occurs flip your pancakes.

7. Continue cooking until the middle has been well cooked. Check with your fork.

8. Add to your plate along with your Greek yogurt.

9. Serve!

Nutritional Value

275 Calories.

36 grams of Protein.

29 grams of Carbs.

1 gram of Fat.

Pumpkin Cream Cheese Pancakes (Serves 1)

Ingredients:

Pancakes:

2 Eggs

2 tablespoons of Coconut Flour

2 ounces of Cream Cheese

1/4 tablespoon of Pumpkin Pie Spice

Pumpkin Butter:

3 tablespoons of Unsalted Butter

1/16 teaspoon of Raw Stevia

1/2 tablespoon of 100% Pumpkin

Directions:

1. Mix together your pumpkin and butter. Microwave for intervals of 10 seconds until it is smooth. Once it's smooth, add in your Stevia for taste.

2. Next work on pancakes. Mix your eggs, cream cheese, pumpkin pie spice, and coconut flour until blended together.

3. Heat your non-stick pan over a medium heat. Add a tablespoon of butter.

4. When your butter begins to brown add in half of your pancake mix.

5. Once your edges brown or the center bubbles, flip your pancake.

6. Cook for around 1 minute or until the center is cooked. Check with your fork.

7. Remove from your pan and add to your plate.

8. Repeat this process with your next pancake.

9. Once all your pancakes are done add your pumpkin butter.

10. Serve!

Squash Spaghetti Pancakes (Serves 2)

Ingredients:

10 ounces of Cooked Spaghetti Squash

2 Eggs

1 ounce of Parmesan Cheese

4 slices of Thick Cut Bacon

1 teaspoon of Onion Powder

1 teaspoon of Garlic Powder

1 teaspoon of Salt

1 teaspoon of Pepper

Directions:

1. Cook your spaghetti squash.

2. Cook your bacon until it's crispy.

3. Add your eggs, spices, cheese, and spaghetti squash to your bowl and mix.

4. Crumble your bacon and add it to your mixture.

5. Heat your bacon grease in the skillet until they are shimmering.

6. Scoop your mixture into bacon grease. Make four piles and then use a spatula to compress your piles flat.

7. After bottom begins to brown flip it.

8. You can add a dollop of sour cream or some chives if you want.

9. Serve!

Nutritional Value:

287 Calories.

19 grams of Protein.

10 grams of Carbs.

18 grams of Fat.

Keto French Toast (Serves 4)

Ingredients:

8 Large Eggs

3/4 cup of Unsweetened Almond Milk

2 teaspoon of Baking Powder

1/4 cup of Coconut Flour

1 teaspoon of Vanilla Extract

1/4 cup of Melted Butter

1/4 cup of Fresh Whole Butter

1 tablespoon of Swerve or Sugar Equivalent

1/2 cup of Heavy Whipping Cream

Pinch of Salt

Directions:

1. Mix your coconut flour, baking powder, salt, and sugar.

2. In a different bowl, whisk together 4 of your 8 eggs. Add 1/4 cup of your almond milk and vanilla. Whisk together.

3. Add your dry and wet ingredients together and whisk. Continue to do so while pouring in your melted butter.

4. Grease your 12 microwave safe containers. Use wide containers.

5. Microwave your muffins. For each additional muffin add a minute to your microwave time. I made 2 batches of 6 muffins with 6 minutes for each batch.

6. While your muffins are cooking, in your large-sized mixing bowl, whisk together your other 4 eggs, 1/2 cup of heavy cream, and 1/2 cup of almond milk.

7. As muffins come out of your microwave, pop them out of containers and allow them to cool for a minute. When they are cool enough, add to your egg mixture and allow them to sit for a couple minutes. Flip them occasionally while letting them sit.

8. Once they've absorbed some of your mixture, heat up your large-sized skillet over a medium-low heat. Add some fresh butter and melt it.

9. Fry your muffins like you would French toast.

10. Serve!

Nutritional Value:

491 Calories.

16 grams of Protein.

8 grams of Carbs.

44 grams of Fat.

Crunchy Keto Cereal w/ Strawberries

Ingredients:

1 package of Bob's Red Mill Flaked Coconut

2 medium sized Strawberries

Unsweetened Almond Milk

Stevia

Ground Cinnamon

Parchment Paper or Coconut Oil

Directions:

1. Preheat your oven to 350 degrees.

2. Line your cookie sheet with your parchment paper. If no parchment paper grease your cooking sheet using coconut oil.

3. Pour your coconut flakes on your cookie sheet.

4. Cook in your oven for approximately 5 minutes.

5. Shuffle flakes around and continue cooking until they are a lightly toasted and lightly tan.

6. Take your flakes out of your oven.

7. Sprinkle them lightly with cinnamon. Can also sprinkle lightly with Stevia.

8. Throw your toasted chips in your bowl and pour your almond milk over them.

9. Slice up 2 strawberries as the garnish on top.

10. Serve!

Chapter Two: Ketogenic Diet Lunch Recipes

In this section, I will give you 30+ keto lunch recipes you can make yourself. I'll include both basic recipes and a few more advanced recipes. That way no matter what your level is in the kitchen you'll be able to prepare yourself a healthy low-carb ketogenic meal to keep you on track with your diet. I'll add in the nutritional value whenever possible, although I don't always have those exact numbers for each and every recipe.

Berry & Chicken Summer Salad (Serves 2)

Ingredients:

1 Chicken Breast

3/4 cup of Blueberries

6 Diced Strawberries

3 tablespoons of Raspberry Balsamic Vinegar

2 cups of Spinach

1/2 cup of Chopped Walnuts

3 tablespoons of Crumbled Feta Cheese

Directions:

1. Cut your chicken breast up into small-sized cubes and cook in your pan. When done place on your plate to cool off.

2. Gather your other ingredients and add them to your large-sized bowl. Add your dressing.

3. Add your chicken and toss your salad.

4. Serve!

Nutritional Value:

335 Calories.

21 grams of Protein.

16 grams of Carbs.

19 grams of Fat.

Grilled Halloumi Salad (Serves 1)

Ingredients:

5 Grape Tomatoes

1 Persian Cucumber

1/2 ounce of Chopped Walnuts

3 ounces of Halloumi Cheese

Handful of Baby Arugula

Olive Oil

Balsamic Vinegar

Salt

Directions:

1. Cut your halloumi cheese into approximately 1/3-inch sized slices.

2. Grill your slices for approximately 3 to 5 minutes on both sides. Should have nice grill marks on each side.

3. Prep your salad by washing then cutting your vegetables. Cut your tomatoes in half and cut your cucumbers into smaller slices. Chop your walnuts and add them in your salad bowl.

4. Wash your baby arugula and add to your bowl.

5. Arrange your grilled halloumi cheese on top of your salad. Add some salt. Dress your salad with your balsamic vinegar and olive oil.

6. Serve!

Nutritional Value:

560 Calories.

21 grams of Protein.

7 grams of Carbs.

47 grams of Fat.

Keto Mini Chicken Pot Pies (Serves 12)

Ingredients:

Filling:

1 pound of Diced Chicken Breast

1 Medium Diced Onion

2 tablespoons of Butter

1/2 cup of Coarsely Grated Carrot

2 stalks of Finely Chopped Celery

1 tablespoon of White Wine Vinegar

1/4 teaspoon of Dried Thyme Leaves

1 1/2 cups of Heavy Cream

1/2 cup of Chicken Stock

2 teaspoons of Paprika

1/2 cup of Fresh or Frozen Green Peas

Salt

Pepper

Crust:

2 Large Eggs

1 cup of Almond Flour

1/2 cup of Coconut Flour

10 tablespoons of Butter

2 teaspoons of Baking Powder

3 cups of Part-Skim Mozzarella Cheese (Grated)

1/4 teaspoon of Dried Thyme

1/4 teaspoon of Sea Salt

Directions:

1. Preheat your oven to 350 degrees. If you're using a metal pan instead of a silicone cupcake/muffin pan, grease it lightly. Place your pan on your cookie sheet. Have 2 sheets of parchment paper about 16-inches long and a rolling pin handy.

2. Begin by preparing your filling. Over a medium-high heat melt 1 tablespoon of butter in your large-sized skillet. When your butter stops foaming add your diced chicken.

3. Brown your chicken on all sides, then sprinkle lightly with your salt and pepper. Turn the heat to low and continue cooking until your chicken is cooked throughout. Remove your chicken to a plate and set to the side for later.

4. Heat your same skillet to medium and add 1 tablespoon of butter. When your butter has stopped foaming add your onions, dried thyme, celery, and to your skillet. Cook, stirring frequently until your onions are slightly brown on the edges and cooked through.

5. Add your white wine vinegar and stir, scraping up any browned bits. When your vinegar becomes syrupy add the broth. Turn the heat to high until your broth simmers, then turn to low and simmer broth and vegetables until broth is reduced and slightly thickened.

6. Stir in your cream and paprika. Simmer on low until thickened.

7. Add your chicken, peas, and any drippings into the sauce and briefly reheat. Sprinkle to taste with your salt and pepper. Turn off your heat and set to the side until your crust is ready to fill.

8. Add your almond flour, coconut flour, baking powder, salt and, dried thyme to your medium-sized mixing bowl. Mix thoroughly using your whisk.

9. Break eggs into your small-sized bowl. Whisk to break up your yolks. Add your eggs to your dry ingredients and stir. A silicone scraper works well for this process. The mixture will be mealy.

10. Place your large-sized saucepan over a low heat. Add your butter and mozzarella cheese. Stir constantly until your butter and cheese are melted. Do not be concerned if they remain separated.

11. When both your cheese and butter are melted, remove from the heat and add your flour and egg mix, stirring rapidly. They do not have to combine completely.

12. Pour your mixture out onto one of the pieces of parchment paper. While your dough is hot (but not hot enough to burn hands), knead it to completely mix in your flour mixture. Form your dough into a log shape and divide into 1/3 and 2/3 parts.

13. Working quickly, cut your larger section of dough into 12 equal sections. Roll each section between 2 pieces of parchment paper to about a 4 1/2-inch circle. Press each circle into your cup on your muffin tin.

14. Roll out the remaining third of your dough. Using your biscuit cutter, cut out 12 circles to function as the top crust. It will be necessary to take the bits of dough not cut into circles and re-roll to cut more circles.

15. Spoon your filling evenly into the bottom crust in the muffin cups. Do not over-fill. If you have extra filling, serve it with the pot pies to pour over the top.

16. Top each of your mini pot pies with a circle and pinch the edges to seal. Flute edges if desired. Using the point of a sharp knife, poke two to four vents in the top. Place your muffin tin on your cookie sheet.

17. Bake your pot pies in your preheated oven for about 17 to 22 minutes or until the tops are a golden brown.

18. Allow it to cool on the rack for about 5 minutes before removing them from your muffin pan.

19. Serve!

Nutritional Value:

445 Calories.

23 grams of Protein.

6 grams of Carbs.

36 grams of Fat.

Keto Kale & Sausage Soup (Serves 6)

Ingredients:

1 pound of Sweet Italian Sausage (Ground)

1 Medium Carrot (Peeled & Diced)

1 Medium Yellow Onion (Chopped)

1 tablespoon of Butter

2 cloves of Crushed Garlic

1 teaspoon of Dried Oregano

2 tablespoons of Red Wine Vinegar

1 teaspoon of Dried Rubbed Sage

1 teaspoon of Dried Basil

1/2 teaspoon of Crushed Red Pepper Flakes

1 cup of Heavy Whipping Cream

4 cups of Low-Sodium Chicken Broth

3 cups of Chopped Kale

1/2 Medium Head Cauliflower (Cut Into Small Florets)

1 teaspoon of Sea Salt

1/2 teaspoon of Freshly Ground Black Pepper

Directions:

1. Heat your large-sized saucepan or Dutch oven over a medium-high heat. Add your ground sausage, breaking up your meat. Cook, stirring occasionally until browned and cooked through, Should take approximately 5 minutes.

2. Using your slotted spoon, remove your cooked sausage and allow to drain on a plate covered with your paper towels. Discard the drippings, but do not wash your pan.

3. Melt your butter over a medium heat. When the bubbling subsides, add your onion and carrot. Cook until your onion begins to brown on the edges and becomes somewhat translucent.

4. Stir your garlic into your onion and carrot mixture. Cook for approximately 1 minute. Add your red wine vinegar and cook until syrupy, scraping up any browned bits. Should take about 1 minute.

5. Stir in your oregano, basil, sage and red pepper flakes. Pour in your stock and heavy cream. Increase the heat to a medium high.

6. When your soup reaches a simmer, add your cauliflower and turn the heat down to a medium-low. Simmer uncovered until your cauliflower is fork-tender. Should take about 10 minutes. Stir in your kale and cooked sausage. Cook 1 to 2 minutes longer, or until your kale wilts and your sausage is reheated.

7. Season with your salt and pepper. The amount of salt needed may vary due to variation in brands of broth.

8. Serve!

Nutritional Value:

298 Calories.

16 grams of Protein.

6 grams of Carbs.

24 grams of Fat.

Apple & Ham Flatbread (Serves 8)

Ingredients:

Crust:

2 cups of Part-Skim Mozzarella Cheese (Grated)

2 tablespoons of Cream Cheese

3/4 cup of Almond Flour

1/8 teaspoon of Dried Thyme

1/2 teaspoon of Sea Salt

Topping:

1 cup of Mexican Cheese (Grated)

4 ounces of Low Carbohydrate Sliced Ham (Cut Into Chunks)

1/4 Medium Apple (Seeded, Cored, & Unpeeled)

1/2 Small Red Onion (Cut Into Thin Slices)

1/8 teaspoon of Dried Thyme

Salt

Pepper

Directions:

1. Preheat your oven to 425 degrees. Cut 2 pieces of parchment paper about 2-inches larger than your 12-inch pizza pan. Have your rolling pin and a 12-inch pizza pan ready.

2. Prepare your double boiler. A sauce pot partially filled with water with your mixing bowl that fits on top will suffice. Over a high heat, bring your water in the pot to a simmer, then turn the heat to low.

3. In your mixing bowl for the double boiler, add your mozzarella cheese, cream cheese, almond flour, thyme, and salt. Place your bowl over the simmering pot and stir constantly being careful not to burn yourself with the steam escaping between your bowl and the pot. A silicone mitt works well to hold the bowl.

4. When your cheese melts enough that your ingredients hold together and it starts to resemble dough, dump it out onto one of the prepared pieces of parchment. Knead for a few minutes to mix your dough thoroughly.

5. Roll your dough into a ball, then place onto the center of your parchment paper. Pat into a disk shape and cover with the other piece of parchment. Using your rolling pin, gently roll your dough into about a 12-inch circle. If the bottom parchment paper rumples, turn your dough over and straighten the parchment paper before continuing.

6. Place your dough and the bottom piece of your parchment onto the pizza pan. Using your fork, poke holes all over the dough. Place your pan in the oven and bake for approximately 6 to 8 minutes, watching carefully. Remove when it is golden brown. Decrease your oven setting to 350 degrees.

7. Sprinkle 1/4 cup of your cheese over the flatbread.

8. Arrange your onion slices.

9. Add your apple slices.

10. Layer on your ham pieces.

11. Cover with your remaining 3/4 cup of cheese. Sprinkle with your thyme, salt, and ground pepper.

12. Bake at 350 degrees until your cheese is melted and the crust is golden brown. Should take about 5 to 7 minutes.

13. Remove your apple and ham flatbread from your oven and slide off of the parchment onto your cooling rack. Allow to cool for 2 to 3 minutes before cutting. Transfer to your cutting board and slice it into 8 pieces.

14. Serve!

Nutritional Value:

255 Calories.

16 grams of Protein.

4 grams of Carbs.

20 grams of Fat.

Broccoli Chicken Zucchini Boats (Serves 2)

Ingredients:

6 ounces of Shredded Rotisserie Chicken

3 ounces of Shredded Cheddar Cheese

2 Large Zucchini (Hollowed Out)

2 tablespoons of Sour Cream

2 tablespoons of Butter

1 stalk of Green Onion

1 cup of Broccoli

Salt

Pepper

Directions:

1. Preheat your oven to 400 degrees and cut your zucchini in half lengthwise. The longer the zucchini the better for this specific recipe.

2. Using your spoon, scoop out most of the zucchini until you're left with a shell about 1 centimeter thick.

3. Pour 1 tablespoon of melted butter into each zucchini boat. Season with your salt and pepper and place them in your oven. This allows your zucchini to cook down while you prepare the filling. This should take approximately 20 minutes.

4. Shred your rotisserie chicken using two forks to pull your meat apart. Measure out 6 ounces and save the rest for another meal.

5. Cut up your broccoli florets until they're bite sized.

6. Combine your chicken and broccoli with your sour cream to keep them moist and creamy. Season in this step as well.

7. Once your zucchini has had a chance to cook, take them out and add your chicken and broccoli filling.

8. Sprinkle your cheddar cheese over the top of your chicken and broccoli and pop them back into your oven for an additional 10 to 15 minutes or until your cheese is melted and browning.

9. Garnish with your chopped green onion and enjoy with sour cream or mayo if so desired.

10. Serve!

Nutritional Value:

476 Calories.

30 grams of Protein.

5 grams of Carbs.

34 grams of Fat.

Bacon, Avocado, & Chicken Sandwich (Serves 2)

Ingredients:

3 Large Eggs

1/8 teaspoon of Cream of Tartar

3 ounces of Cream Cheese

1/2 teaspoon of Garlic Powder

1/4 teaspoon of Salt

Filling:

3 ounces of Chicken

1 tablespoon of Mayonnaise

2 slices of Pepper Jack Cheese

1 teaspoon of Sriracha

1/4 Medium Avocado

2 slices of Bacon

2 Grape Tomatoes

Directions:

1. Preheat your oven to 300 degrees. Begin separating your 3 eggs into to 2 dry bowls.

2. Add your cream of tartar and salt to your egg whites. Using an electric mixer, whip your egg whites until you see soft, foamy peaks form.

3. In your other bowl, combine 3 ounces of cubed cream cheese with your egg yolks and beat until a pale yellow color.

4. Gently fold your egg whites into your yolks, half at a time.

5. On your parchment paper lined baking sheet, spoon about 1/4 cup of your bread batter.

6. Using your spatula, press gently on tops of the bread to form squares. Then sprinkle the tops with your garlic powder and bake for approximately 25 minutes.

7. While your bread is baking, cook your chicken and bacon with some salt and pepper.

8. To arrange your sandwich, begin by combining mayo and sriracha and spreading that onto the underside of one pieces of bread. Add your chicken onto your mayo mixture.

9. Add 2 slices of pepper jack cheese and the bacon, nestle some of your halved grape tomatoes and spread some mashed avocado on top. Season to taste, and top with the other piece of bread.

Nutritional Value:

361 Calories.

22 grams of Protein.

2 grams of Carbs.

28 grams of Fat.

Simple Chicken Salad (Serves 6)

Ingredients:

4 Chicken Breasts

3 Large Hardboiled Eggs

3.5 ounces of Green Peppers

1 ounce of Green Onions

4.5 ounces of Celery

3/4 cup of Sugar-Free Sweet Relish

3/4 cup of Mayo

Directions:

1. Preheat your oven to 350 degrees.

2. Add your chicken to your oven safe pan.

3. Cook for approximately 45 to 60 minutes until your chicken is finished cooking.

4. Place 3 eggs in your pan and cover them with water. Bring it to a boil and then cook for approximately 15 minutes once your water is boiling.

5. While your chicken is in the oven cooking, chop up your onions, celery, and peppers.

6. Once your chicken is out of your oven allow it to cool down and then chop up.

7. Combine all of your ingredients in your large-sized bowl.

8. Chop up your eggs and mix in. Add your eggs last.

9. Split into 6 separate portions or containers.

10. Serve!

Nutritional Value:

413 Calories.

43 grams of Protein.

2 grams of Carbs.

25 grams of Fat.

Easy Buffalo Wings (Serves 2)

Ingredients:

6 Chicken Wings (6 Drumettes & 6 Wingettes)

1/2 cup of Frank's Red Hot Sauce

2 tablespoons of Butter

Garlic Powder

Paprika

Salt

Pepper

Cayenne (optional)

Directions:

1. Break each of your chicken wings into 2 different pieces. The drumettes and wingettes, getting rid of the tips.

2. Pour your hot sauce over your wings. Enough to lightly coat them.

3. Season your wings with spices and cover them. Place in your refrigerator for 1 hour.

4. Place your broiler on high and put your oven rack 6-inches from your broiler. Put your aluminum paper on your baking sheet. Place your wings on your sheet with enough room so the flames can reach their sides.

5. Cook for approximately 8 minutes under your broiler. Your wings should turn dark brown on top. May turn black if they are close to the flame.

6. Melt your butter on your oven top and add the rest of your hot sauce. Can also add cayenne if you want your wings to be spicier.

7. Once your butter has melted take off of the heat.

8. Take your wings from the broiler and flip them. Cook another 6 to 8 minutes.

9. Once good and browned on all sides take out of your broiler and add to your bowl.

10. Pour butter-hot sauce mixture over your wings. Toss wings to coat evenly.

11. Serve!

Nutritional Value:

620 Calories.

48 grams of Protein.

1 gram of Carbs.

46 grams of Fat.

Oopsie Rolls (Serves 12)

Ingredients:

3 Large Eggs

3 ounces of Cream Cheese

1/8 teaspoon of Cream of Tartar

1/8 teaspoon of Salt

Directions:

1. Preheat your oven to 300 degrees.

2. Separate your eggs from egg yolks. Place each in different bowls.

3. With an electric hand mixer beat your egg whites until they get very bubbly.

4. Add in your cream of tarter. Beat it until a stiff peak has formed.

5. In your egg yolk bowl, add your 3 ounces of cream cheese and salt.

4. Beat your egg yolk mixture until your yolks are a pale looking yellow and they have doubled in their size.

5. Fold your egg whites into the egg yolk mixture. Don't use an electric hand mixer. Gently fold it together.

6. Line your cookie sheet with parchment paper and spray with some oil or grease. Dollop your batter as big as you want them. I make 12 of equal size and the nutritional value amount reflects that.

7. Bake for approximately 30 to 40 minutes. They are done when the tops of your oopsie rolls are firm and golden.

8. Allow them to cool on your wire rack.

9. Serve!

<u>Nutritional Value:</u>

45 Calories.

2.3 grams of Protein.

0 grams of Carbs.

3.8 grams of Fat.

Cucumber Sushi Rolls (Serves 2)

Ingredients:

1/2 pound of Tuna Steak

1/2 Avocado

2 Cucumbers

2 tablespoons of Mayonnaise

8 Shrimp

1/2 teaspoon of Sesame Seeds

2 teaspoons of Sriracha

1 stalk of Green Onion

Directions:

1. Peel your cucumbers and cut off their ends. You want to have two 6 to 8-inch long cylindrical shaped cucumbers when done.

2. Use your wet long knife and lay the edge of it against an edge of your cucumber. Begin cutting into it. Knife should be barely visible under your transparent cucumber.

3. Once your cucumber is cut to its seeds gather your other ingredients.

4. Mix your mayo and sriracha to make spicy mayo.

5. Take the end of your cucumber with your fish and begin rolling it onto itself. Make sure to keep your roll tight so that no air pockets form. The ingredients need to stick to one another, otherwise, they'll fall right out.

6. Once you're almost done rolling it and only have approximately 2 to 3-inches left of your cucumber, spread some of your spicy mayo on your cucumber and finish the roll. The mayonnaise will act as sort of glue to help keep your cucumber sealed.

7. Carefully slice your cucumber into 1/2 inch to 1-inch rounds. Hold both sides of your cucumber as slicing to help maintain its shape.

8. You should now have 6 to 8 pieces of sushi per roll. Chop up your green onion and sprinkle on top.

9. Serve!

Nutritional Value:

322 Calories.

36 grams of Protein.

2.5 grams of Carbs.

17 grams of Fat.

Tuna Tartare (Serves 2)

Ingredients:

1 pound of Tuna Steak

1 Avocado

3 stalks of Scallion

1 teaspoon of Jalapeno

1 tablespoon of Soy Sauce

2 tablespoons of Olive Oil

2 tablespoons of Sesame Seed Oil

1 teaspoon of Sesame Seeds

1 tablespoon of Mayo

1 tablespoon of Sriracha

2 Persian Cucumbers

1/2 Lime

Directions:

1. Dice your tuna steak and your avocado into 1/4-inch cubes. Put them in your bowl.

2. Dice your jalapeno and scallion. Add them to your bowl.

3. Pour your sesame oil, olive oil, soy sauce, mayo, juice from a lime, and sriracha into your bowl.

4. Gently combine your ingredients using your hands.

5. Slice your Persian cucumber and sprinkle with your sesame seeds.

6. Serve!

Nutritional Value:

487 Calories.

56.7 grams of Protein.

4 grams of Carbs.

24.5 grams of Fat.

Simple Cucumber Sandwich (Serves 1)

Ingredients:

1 Cucumber

1.5 ounces of Boursin Cheese

Sliced Meat

Directions:

1. Slice your cucumber into half and use your melon baller to remove any seeds and some of the cucumber itself.

2. Fill the one side with your spreadable Boursin cheese.

3. Fold your sliced deli meat longways so you can fill the other half.

4. Serve!

Nutritional Value: (Will Depend on Type of Deli Meat Used)

196 Calories.

17 grams of Protein.

7 grams of Carbs.

12 grams of Fat.

Avgolemono Soup (Serves 8)

Ingredients:

4 Shredded Chicken Breasts

3 Eggs

6 cups of Chicken Broth

2 Juiced Lemons

2 tablespoons of Olive Oil

1 Medium Onion

1/2 cup of Heavy Cream

1/2 head of Riced Cauliflower

2 cups of Water

Dill

Chopped Parsley

Salt

Pepper

Directions:

1. Rice your head of cauliflower by removing the leaves and chopping them into large-sized florets. Grate your florets on coarsest side of your box grater a few times.

2. Cook your chicken in an oiled pan. Once cooked pull the meat apart until it is in small-sized pieces.

3. In your large oiled pot cook your onions over a medium heat until turning brown and translucent.

4. Add your water, chicken broth, heavy cream, riced cauliflower, and chicken.

5. Add in your herbs and lemon juice. Taste and make sure your soup has lemon flavor and is salted enough to your liking.

6. Cook for approximately 8 minutes until your cauliflower gets tender.

7. While your soup is cooking get your bowl and beat together your eggs in it. While whisking your eggs with your one hand, pour a ladle of your soup broth into your eggs with your other hand slowly so it doesn't cook the eggs unevenly.

8. When your eggs have 1 to 2 ladles full of the soup broth in them turn the flame under your pot off.

9. Pour your egg mixture into the soup slowly, stirring your soup while pouring.

10. Don't turn the heat back on. Allow the soup to bring your eggs to their full temperature for approximately 2 to 3 minutes.

11. Add some pepper and chopped parsley.

12. Serve!

Nutritional Value:

251 Calories.

20.7 grams of Protein.

5.3 grams of Carbs.

16.3 grams of Fat.

Buffalo Chicken Soup (Serves 4)

Ingredients:

4 Chicken Breasts

6 tablespoons of Butter

2 Carrots

2 ounces of Cream Cheese

4 stalks of Celery

1/2 cup of Frank's Red Hot Sauce

1 quart of Chicken Broth

1/2 teaspoon of Cayenne

1/2 cup of Heavy Cream

1/2 teaspoon of Thyme

1 teaspoon of Salt

Directions:

1 Set your celery and carrot to cook in your oiled pot.

2. When they've begun to break down put in your chicken breast to cook with them. Cover your pot to let them steam and cook faster.

3. Once your chicken is fully cooked remove from your pot. By cooking your chicken this way it lets a slight crust begin to form around it that boiling wouldn't be able to achieve. Once it's cooked shred your chicken.

4. Pour your chicken broth over your vegetables. Add in your cream cheese, heavy cream, and butter.

5. While that's coming to a boil place your now shredded chicken back into your soup.

6. Add your hot sauce.

7. Add all of your herbs. Let your soup simmer for approximately 15 to 20 minutes. This will allow your flavors to marry.

8. Garnish your soup however you'd like. I prefer using green onion and cold sour cream.

9. Serve!

Nutritional Value:

563 Calories.

57 grams of Protein.

4 grams of Carbs.

32.5 grams of Fat.

Seafood Soup (Serves 6)

Ingredients:

Soup:

10 ounces of Wild Caught Cod

8 ounces of Calamari

8 ounces of Shrimp

1/3 cup of Coconut Oil

1 1/2 cups of Tomato Sauce

1 quart of Seafood Broth

1/2 cup of Coconut Cream

1 Medium Onion

3 Medium Carrots

4 stalks of Green Onion

2 cups of Water

8 ounces of Mushrooms

4 stalks of Celery

4 cloves of Garlic

1 Lemon

1 Lime

Spices:

2 teaspoons of Red Pepper Flakes

1 teaspoon of Dill

1 teaspoon of Thyme

2 teaspoons of Basil

3 Whole Bay Leaves

2 teaspoons of Oregano

2 teaspoons of Pepper

1 tablespoon of Salt

Fresh Parsley

Directions:

1. Start with 2 tablespoons of coconut oil in your soup pot over a medium flame.

2. Throw in your crushed garlic and onions. Cook them until they are fragrant.

3. Throw in your chopped celery and carrots. Allow them to cook until they are tender.

4. Pour in 1 quart of broth, tomato sauce, and water.

5. Allow it to come to boil. Reduce your heat to a simmer. Allow your vegetables and broth to simmer for approximately 30 minutes. Season with your salt and pepper.

6. While your soup is still simmering, peel your shrimp. Set to the side.

7. Cut your calamari tubes into 1/2-inch pieces and set them in your bowl with lemon juice.

8. Chop your mushrooms up and add to your soup after the soup has been simmering for around 30 minutes. Add your coconut cream. Make sure your soup returns to a simmer if your cream cooled off the soup too much.

9. Once your mushrooms have cooked for approximately 10 minutes add in your cod and cook for another 10 minutes.

10. Break your fish down in your pot using your wooden spoon to break it into smaller-sized pieces.

11. Make sure your water is simmering before cooking your shrimp. Turn the heat up a little bit and add your shrimp. Cook for approximately 3 minutes.

12. After approximately 3 minutes add in your calamari to the soup. Don't add in lemon juice. Allow it to cook for 2 more minutes. Any longer and your calamari may get rubbery and the shrimp might start getting hard.

13. Take your pot off the heat. Add in your lime juice. Top with your fresh parsley and chopped green onion. Remove your bay leaves.

14. Serve!

Nutritional Value:

284 Calories.

27 grams of Protein.

9 grams of Carbs.

14 grams of Fat.

*

Chili Chicken Soup (Serves 8)

Ingredients:

8 Boneless Chicken Thighs

1 Onion

1 Pepper

2 tablespoons of Unsalted Butter

8 slices of Bacon

1/4 cup of Unsweetened Coconut Milk

1 tablespoon of Thyme

1 tablespoon of Minced Garlic

3 tablespoons of Tomato Paste

1 tablespoon of Coconut Flour

3 tablespoons of Lemon Juice

1 cup of Chicken Stock

1 teaspoon of Pepper

1 teaspoon of Salt

Directions:

1. Put a pat of your butter in the center of your crockpot.

2. Slice your peppers and onions thinly. Distribute them evenly over the bottom of your crockpot.

3. Cover them with your boneless chicken thighs.

4. Cut up your bacon and place over your chicken.

5. Add your coconut flour, pepper, salt, and garlic.

6. Add your liquids (chicken stock, lemon juice, and coconut milk).

7. Add your tomato paste.

8. Cook on low for approximately 6 hours.

9. Stir and break up your chicken.

10. Serve!

Nutritional Value:

396 Calories.

41 grams of Protein.

7 grams of Carbs.

21 grams of Fat.

Bacon Cheddar Cauliflower Soup (Serves 6)

Ingredients:

4 slices of Bacon

1 Medium Onion

1 Cauliflower Head

12 ounces of Aged Cheddar

2 tablespoons of Olive Oil

3 cups of Chicken Broth

1 teaspoon of Ground Thyme

1 tablespoon of Minced Garlic

1/4 cup of Heavy Cream

1 ounce of Parmesan Cheese

Directions:

1. Dice your cauliflower and place on your foil lined baking sheet. Drizzle it with your olive oil.

2. Separately pepper and salt your cauliflower and bacon. Cook your cauliflower for approximately 35 minutes at 375 degrees.

3. Cook your bacon until it is crisp.

4. In a large-sized pot that will fit your soup, dice your medium onion and fry it up in your bacon grease.

5. Once your onion is cooked, add your thyme and garlic and cook for between 30 seconds and 1 minute.

6. Add your cauliflower and chicken broth. Simmer while covered for approximately 20 minutes.

7. While your cauliflower simmers, shred your aged cheddar.

8. Using your immersion blender, blend your cauliflower into your soup.

9. Add your cheese and blend some more.

10. Add your cream and bacon. Mix together with your spoon.

11. Serve!

Nutritional Value:

337 Calories.

18 grams of Protein.

11 grams of Carbs.

25 grams of Fat.

Easy Lobster Bisque (Serves 4)

Ingredients:

24 ounces of Lobster Chunks

2 Carrots

1/2 Red Onion

1/2 cup of Tomato Paste

4 cloves of Garlic

1 tablespoon of Olive Oil

3 Bay Leaves

1 quart of Seafood Broth

2 cups of White Wine

4 stalks of Celery

1 ounce of Brandy

1 teaspoon of Peppercorns

1 cup of Heavy Cream

1 teaspoon of Paprika

1 teaspoon of Thyme

1 teaspoon of Xanthan Gum

1 tablespoon of Fresh Lemon Juice

1 tablespoon of Salt

Parsley

Directions:

1. Chop your garlic, carrots, celery, and onion.

2. In your soup pot cook your onion in olive oil until fragrant. Add your garlic and cook until your pan starts looking black and crusty at the bottom.

3. Deglaze your pot using white wine. Add your carrot and celery.

4. Pour in broth, tomato paste, and brandy. Stir to help incorporate.

5. Add your spices and let your soup simmer for 60 minutes.

6. Once your soup is cooked remove and discard your bay leaves.

7. Add your cream and allow your soup to come to a simmer.

8. Add in a small portion of xanthan gum slowly while stirring your soup. Should see your soup thicken.

9. Pour your soup into your blender. Blend soup before adding lobster chunks. If you want a chunkier bisque don't blend at all. If blending continue to do so until it is creamy.

10. If your lobster isn't cooked, cut into chunks and saute in some olive oil and butter in your pan.

11. Pour your bisque into a bowl and add your lobster chunks. Stir well until it is combined.

12. Dress your bisque with some green onion, lemon juice, and parsley.

13. Serve!

Nutritional Value:

220 Calories.

12 grams of Protein.

8 grams of Carbs.

15 grams of Fat.

Simple Clam Chowder (Serves 4)

Ingredients:

3 strips of Bacon

1 Carrot

2 tablespoons of Butter

1 Onion

1 cup of Clam Juice

16 ounces of Canned Clams

2 stalks of Celery

2 1/2 cups of Heavy Cream

4 cloves of Garlic

1 teaspoon of Xanthan Gum

1 cup of Water

1 teaspoon of Parsley

1/2 a head of Cauliflower

1/2 teaspoon of Celery Salt

1/2 teaspoon of Thyme

1 teaspoon of Pepper

1 teaspoon of Salt

Directions:

1. Set your pot of water to a boil.

2. Cut half a head of your cauliflower into medium-size florets. Throw your cauliflower into the water once boiling and cook for approximately 10 minutes. They should get very soft by the time they're done.

3. While your cauliflower boils, chop your other ingredients. Bacon should be in 1/2-inch cubed pieces. Carrot and onion should be minced. Celery should be cut into slices that are a 1/4-inch.

4. Throw your bacon in your large-sized soup pot on a medium heat and cook until it is crispy. Once your bacon is cooked, add in your onion, celery, and carrot. Sprinkle with a little salt and cook until your onion begins to turn translucent.

5. Add in some butter and squeezed garlic.

6. Open your canned clams and separate juice by putting your strainer in a bowl and pouring canned clams in. Save both juice and the clams.

7. By now your cauliflower should be done. Drain your water and put them into your blender or a Nutribullet with a bit of water. Blend them until they are creamy.

8. Add your blended cauliflower, water, clam juice, heavy cream, and vegetables to the bacon. Lower the flame to a low heat and allow to simmer for approximately 20 minutes.

9. Spice your chowder with celery salt, pepper, salt. Add your thyme last.

10. Add in your xanthan gum.

11. Add your clams. Cook your clams until warmed up. Should be approximately 5 minutes at the most. Overcooking the clams will leave them tough and very chewy.

12. Sprinkle some thyme on top of your chowder.

13. Serve!

Nutritional Value:

804 Calories.

28 grams of Protein.

15 grams of Carbs.

66 grams of Fat.

Easy Beef Stew (Serves 6)

Ingredients:

5 pounds of Beef Shank

2 Medium Onions

3 Medium Carrots

8 cloves of Garlic

8 Campari Tomatoes

2 tablespoons of Apple Cider Vinegar

2 cups of Water

1/4 cup of Tomato Sauce

1 quart of Chicken Broth

Spices:

3 teaspoons of Crushed Red Pepper

2 teaspoons of Basil

2 teaspoons of Onion Powder

3 Whole Bay Leaves

2 teaspoons of Parsley

1 teaspoon of Cayenne

2 teaspoons of Garlic Powder

4 teaspoons of Salt

2 teaspoons of Black Pepper

Directions:

1. Place your cast iron skill on a medium heat while you chop your tomatoes, onion, carrots, and garlic into chunky sized pieces.

2. Place your garlic, carrots, and onions into a soup pot that's been oiled or a Dutch oven. Cook until your onions are translucent.

3. In your hot cast iron skillet sear each side of all your beef shanks until a deep brown crust has formed. You're not cooking the beef now, just letting it develop a nice crust that you couldn't get by boiling.

4. Pour your chicken broth over your carrots, onions, and garlic. Add your water and apple cider vinegar.

5. Add your tomatoes, spices, and tomato sauce. Stir it well.

6. When your beef shanks are seared, submerge them each into your broth and allow it to boil.

7. After your stew has come to boil, reduce your heat to a simmer. Allow it to simmer uncovered slightly for approximately 3 hours. Cook until meat is completely cooked and tender.

8. Remove your bay leaves.

9. Serve!

Nutritional Value:

531 Calories.

68 grams of Protein.

9 grams of Carbs.

22 grams of Fat.

Roasted Brussels Sprouts w/ Bacon (Serves 4)

Ingredients:

1 pound of Brussels Sprouts

8 strips of Bacon

2 tablespoons of Olive Oil

Salt

Pepper

Directions:

1. Preheat your oven to 375 degrees. Cut off ends of each of your brussels sprouts. Then cut them down into halves.

2. Put in your large-sized bowl and mix with your salt, pepper, olive oil, and other spice you prefer to use. Sometimes I add red pepper.

3. Pour out onto your greased baking sheet. Leave some room between them.

4. Bake in your oven for approximately 30 minutes. About halfway in, grab your sheet in the oven and give a strong shake so that they rotate a bit.

5. Fry up your bacon while your brussels sprouts are cooking. I do 2 slices per serving.

6. Once your bacon is cooked, chop it into small pieces about 1/2-inch big.

7. Once your brussels sprouts have blackened and shriveled a little they are ready. Take out of your oven and put into your bowl with your bacon. Toss it together and sprinkle some salt on top.

8. Serve!

Nutritional Value:

278 Calories.

15 grams of Protein.

4 grams of Carbs.

21 grams of Fat.

Bacon Cheesy Wrapped Hot Dogs (Serves 4)

Ingredients:

8 strips of Bacon

16 slices of Pepper Jack Cheese

8 Sausage Links

Garlic Powder

Onion Powder

Paprika

Black Pepper

Toothpicks

Directions:

1. Preheat your oven to 400 degrees.

2. Cook your sausage links on your grill or oiled pan until nearly done. Take off the heat and allow it to cool until you can handle them.

3. Cut slits in the middle of each one until they are butterflied. The deeper the cut, the more cheese will fit.

4. Take 2 slices of your cheese and place into the middle of each of your sausage links.

5. Tightly wrap each link in bacon. Secure it with your wet toothpick.

6. Sprinkle on your spices and bake until your bacon gets crispy. Should take approximately 15 to 20 minutes. I suggest flipping them halfway through.

7. Remove from your oven.

8. Serve!

Nutritional Value:

570 Calories.

40 grams of Protein.

4 grams of Carbs.

41 grams of Fat.

Spicy & Sweet Chicken & Shrimp (Serves 2)

Ingredients:

20 Large Shrimped (De-Veined & Peeled)

2 Boneless Chicken Breasts

1/2 pound of Mushrooms

1/4 cup of Mayo

2 tablespoons of Sriracha

2 teaspoons of Lime Juice

1 teaspoon of Garlic Powder

1 tablespoon of Coconut Oil

1/2 teaspoon of Paprika

1/2 teaspoon of Erythritol

1/2 teaspoon of Crushed Red Pepper

1 stalk of Green Onion

2 handfuls of Spinach

1/4 teaspoon of Xanthan Gum

1 teaspoon of Salt

Directions:

1. Tenderize your chicken breasts.

2. Place your chicken breast on an oiled large-sized pan and cook over a medium-high heat. Season them with your garlic powder and salt. Cook for approximately 8 minutes before flipping. Reduce your heat and cover it when flipped onto its other side.

3. Slice your mushrooms and throw them into pan around your chicken as it's cooking. Season them with your garlic powder and salt. Add more oil if necessary.

4. In a separate pan, cook your shrimp and sauce. Get your shrimp ready for cooking. Make sure your shrimp are peeled and deveined.

5. Combine your sriracha, mayo, xanthan gum, and erythritol. Whisk quickly and well.

6. Heat your pan over a medium heat. Lay out your shrimp in an even layer. Quickly combine your shrimp and sauce. Toss completely to coat each of your shrimp. Cook for approximately 3 minutes while stirring often.

7. Once your shrimp are done, turn off the heat and remove your pan. Add your lime juice and toss them again.

8. Prepare a spinach bed and add your cooked mushrooms on top of it.

9. Place your chicken on top of a spinach bed and top it with as much shrimp as you want.

10. Garnish with your green onion and some lime wedges.

11. Serve!

Nutritional Value:

591 Calories.

50 grams of Protein.

3 grams of Carbs.

39 grams of Fat.

Coconut Shrimp (Serves 2)

Ingredients:

Shrimp:

12 Large Shrimp

1 Egg Yolk

1/2 ounce of Flaked Coconut

1 ounce of Shredded Coconut

3 tablespoons of Unsweetened Coconut Milk

6 tablespoons of Mayo

Dip:

4 tablespoons of Mayonnaise

2 teaspoons of Chili Garlic Sauce

1 teaspoon of Unsweetened Lime Juice

Directions:

1. Thaw out and dry your shrimp.

2. Mix the rest of your shrimp ingredients together.

3. Coat your shrimp in this mixture.

4. Drop your shrimp into your fryer and cook until they are golden brown.

5. Mix together all your dip ingredients.

6. Serve!

Nutritional Value:

670 Calories.

11 grams of Protein.

7 grams of Carbs.

69 grams of Fat.

Brussels Sprouts Burgers (Serves 14)

Ingredients:

32 ounces of Brussels Sprouts

3 Eggs

1 1/2 ounces of Green Onion

8 ounces of Parmesan Cheese

1/3 cup of Almond Flour

11 ounces of Goat Cheese

Salt

Pepper

Directions:

1. Wash your brussels sprouts and shred them using your grater setting on your food processor.

2. Finely grate your Parmesan cheese and mix with your brussels sprouts, almond flour, pepper, and salt.

3. Crumble your goat cheese into your mixture and combine with your hands.

4. Beat your 3 eggs together and combine with the rest of your mixture.

5. Patty out 4-ounce Brussels Sprouts burgers.

6. Heat your oil in a cast iron skillet.

7. Fry your burgers for 2 1/2 minutes on each side until crisp.

8. Serve!

Nutritional Value:

182 Calories.

14 grams of Protein.

7 grams of Carbs.

11 grams of Fat.

Keto Quarter Pounder (Serves 2)

Ingredients:

1/2 pound of Ground Beef

1 Egg

1 strip of Bacon

1 tablespoon of Sliced Pickled Jalapenos

1/2 Plum Tomato

1 tablespoon of Mayo

1/4 Onion

1 tablespoon of Sriracha

2 tablespoons of Butter

2 Leaves of Lettuce

Spices:

1/2 teaspoon of Crushed Red Pepper

1/4 teaspoon of Cayenne

1/2 teaspoon of Basil

1/2 teaspoon of Salt

Directions:

1. Knead your meat for approximately 3 minutes.

2. Chop and dice your ingredients finely.

3. Add your bacon, eggs, tomato, 1 tablespoon of butter, and spices together to meat and knead your meat again.

4. Split your meat in half 2 times and flatten all 4 pieces of your meat to make flat-sized patties. Add a tablespoon of butter to the center of 2 pieces of meat and then put on your non-buttered pieces. Seal up their sides so you get 2 big patties that are ready for grilling.

5. Put your patties on the grill. Throw your onions on your grill after flipping burgers at the 5-minute mark.

6. Flip your onions after 2 1/2 minutes to cook evenly on both sides. Cook your burger for an additional 5 minutes. Total cook time for your burger is approximately 10 minutes.

7. Place your patties on 2 big leaves of lettuce and place on your mayo. Top with whatever toppings you prefer. I prefer sriracha and sliced jalapenos.

8. Serve!

Nutritional Value:

443 Calories.

25 grams of Protein.

4 grams of Carbs.

34 grams of Fat.

Sloppy Joe's (Serves 2)

Ingredients:

Meat:

1 pound of Ground Beef

3 strips of Bacon (Chopped)

1/2 cup of Chopped Onion

3 Plum Tomatoes

3 cloves of Garlic

2 tablespoons of Sriracha

1/4 cup of Ketchup

1 teaspoon of Dark Brown Sugar

1 teaspoon of Lemon Juice

1/2 teaspoon of Soy Sauce

2 tablespoons of Mustard

1/2 teaspoon of White Vinegar

Spices:

1 teaspoon of Salt

Dash of Cayenne

Dash of Thyme

Dash of Garlic Powder

Dash of Crushed Red Pepper

Dash of Basil

For Sandwich:

2 Pretzel Buns

1 tablespoon of Butter

1 Sliced Jalapeno

1/2 cup of Shredded Pepper Jack

Directions:

1. Chop up your bacon and onion. Throw your bacon in your hot pan over a medium heat and spread out so it all cooks the same. Once your bacon is browned and your pan is oiled up nicely with your bacon grease, throw in your onion and cook until it is translucent.

2. Place a pot of water to boil. Just enough to cover 2 tomatoes. Once boiling, throw in your tomatoes and boil for approximately 2 minutes. Take out of the water and allow it to cool.

3. Remove your tomato skins. Crush your tomatoes into a pulp and then squeeze your garlic into them.

4. Once your onions are translucent, add your ground beef and begin breaking it into smallish chunks. Lower the flame and allow it to simmer so nothing gets overcooked.

5. Add in your crushed tomato and stir well.

6. Add in your spices, sugar, sriracha, mustard, ketchup, vinegar, soy sauce, and lemon juice. Stir it well and continue to let it simmer.

7. Shred your pepper jack cheese.

8. Cut your pretzel buns in half. In a different pan, melt your butter until it is browned. Place your buns with their flat side down on the butter to soak it and get toasted.

9. Once your Sloppy Joe mixture is cooked and thicker turn off your heat.

10. Sprinkle your cheese on your bottom bun and add Sloppy Joe. Top with your sliced jalapeno.

11. Serve!

Nutritional Value:

817 Calories.

73 grams of Protein.

18 grams of Carbs.

46 grams of Fat.

Avocado Fries (Serves 3)

Ingredients:

1 Egg

1 1/2 cups of Sunflower Oil

3 Avocados

1 1/2 cups of Almond Meal

1/4 teaspoon of Cayenne Pepper

1/2 teaspoon of Salt

Directions:

1. Break your egg into your bowl and beat. In a different bowl, mix your almond meal with cayenne pepper and salt.

2. Slice your avocados in half and remove the seeds.

3. Peel the skin off of every half.

4. Slice your avocado vertically into 4 pieces.

5. Heat deep fryer to 350 degrees.

6. Coat each slice of your avocado in your egg mixture. Roll each coated slice in your almond meal mix.

7. Carefully place each slice into your deep fryer. Do this carefully.

8. Fry for approximately 45 seconds to 1 minute until it is light brown.

9. Quickly transfer to your plate with paper towel on it to soak up your excess oil.

10. Mix your mayo and sriracha sauce.

11. Serve!

Nutritional Value:

587 Calories.

17 grams of Protein.

8 grams of Carbs.

51 grams of Fat.

Portobello Mushroom Pizza (Serves 3)

Ingredients:

3 Portobello Mushrooms

1 1/2 ounces of Monterey Jack

3 slices of Tomato

12 Pepperoni Slices

1 1/2 ounces of Mozzarella

3 teaspoons of Pizza Seasoning

1 1/2 ounces of Cheddar Cheese

9 Spinach Leaves

Drizzle of Olive Oil

Directions:

1. Preheat your convection oven to 450 degrees.

2. De-stem and wash your Portobello mushrooms.

3. Place your mushrooms with cap side down on your foiled lined sheet. Drizzle it with your olive oil.

4. Sprinkle with your pizza seasoning.

5. Layer your spinach, then tomato, then cheese, and a round of seasoning.

6. Cook for approximately 6 minutes until cheese melts.

7. Add your pepperoni and cook until your pepperoni is crispy.

8. Serve!

Nutritional Value:

276 Calories.

19 grams of Protein.

6 grams of Carbs.

21 grams of Fat.

Crispy Chicken Wings (Serves 2)

Ingredients:

12 Raw Chicken Wings

4 tablespoons of Frank's Red Hot

4 tablespoons of Unsalted Butter

Directions:

1. Preheat your fryer oil to 275 degrees.

2. Pat down your wings until it is super dry.

3. Fry your wings for approximately 14 minutes.

4. Allow your wings to rest until they reach room temperature.

5. Preheat your fryer to 375 degrees.

6. Pat your wings dry again.

7. Fry an additional 6 minutes until they are golden brown.

8. Mix in your melted butter and Frank's Red Hot.

9. Toss your wings to coat.

10. Serve!

Nutritional Value:

686 Calories.

42 grams of Protein.

0 grams of Carbs.

55 grams of Fat.

Simple Chicken Nuggets (Serves 2)

Ingredients:

1 Egg

1/2 ounce of Grated Parmesan

4 ounces of Chicken Breast

1/2 teaspoon of Baking Powder

2 tablespoons of Almond Flour

1 tablespoon of Water

Directions:

1. Heat your deep fryer to approximately 375 degrees.

2. Cook your chicken breast. Once cooked cut into cubes.

3. Mix together your almond flour, baking powder, and grated Parmesan.

4. Add your eggs and whisk.

5. Add your water and whisk.

6. Roll your chicken breast in your batter until it is fully coated. Drop them into your frying oil.

7. Make sure they don't stick at the bottom of your fryer. Move them around every minute.

8. Cook for approximately 5 minutes until your batter begins to turn golden brown.

9. Serve!

Nutritional Value:

166 Calories.

3 grams of Protein.

2 grams of Carbs.

8 grams of Fat.

Chapter Three: Ketogenic Diet Dinner Recipes

In this section, I will give you 30+ keto dinner recipes you can make yourself. I'll include both basic recipes and a few more advanced recipes. That way no matter what your level is in the kitchen you'll be able to prepare yourself a healthy low-carb ketogenic meal to keep you on track with your diet. I'll add in the nutritional value whenever possible, although I don't always have those exact numbers for each and every recipe.

Keto Fried Chicken (Serves 10)

Ingredients:

10 pieces of Chicken

3/4 cup of Plain Whey Protein

1 cup of Crushed Pork Rinds

1/2 teaspoon of Onion Powder

1 tablespoon of Oat Fiber

1/2 cup of Parmesan Cheese

2 Large Eggs

1/4 cup of Heavy Cream

1/4 cup of Water

3/4 inch of Deep Hot Oil

1/8 teaspoon of Coarse Black Pepper

Directions:

1. Measure out and then mix together all your dry ingredients in a paper bag. Shake it well.

2. Whisk eggs, water, and cream together in your large-sized bowl.

3. Toss in your pieces of cut up chicken into your egg mix and coat each piece completely.

4. Take pieces out of your bowl and drop in your bag of seasoned flour. When 3 pieces are in your bag, hold the top closed and shake your bag to coat chicken.

5. Heat 3/4-inch deep oil on a high heat.

6. Place your pieces close together. Lower the heat to a medium-high. Brown your chicken on one side. Turn over carefully and brown the opposite side. Should take approximately 30 minutes.

7. Remove and place on your paper towel.

8. Serve!

Keto Chicken Divan (Serves 6)

Ingredients:

2 Boneless Chicken Breasts

3 tablespoons of Ghee

1 Small Yellow Onion

3 cups of Steamed Chopped Broccoli

1/2 tablespoon of Minced Garlic

1 cup of Chicken Stock or Broth

3 cups of Cauliflower

1 teaspoon of Lemon Juice

1/2 cup of Mayonnaise

1 cup of Heavy Cream

2 cups of Shredded Cheddar Cheese

10 cranks of Fresh Pepper

1/2 teaspoon of Garlic Salt

Dash of Parsley

Directions:

1. Preheat your oven to 350 degrees.

2. Fill your pot halfway with water. Add in your chicken breasts.

3. Cook on high heat and bring to a boil until your chicken is cooked.

4. Cook your onions and garlic in a medium frying pan over a low heat with your ghee.

5. While that cooks, blend your cauliflower using your food processor. Do this for a few seconds until it looks like rice.

6. After cooking your onions for 2 minutes, add in your spices one by one mixing each one in.

7. Once your onions are nice and soft, add in your cauliflower.

8. Once your cauliflower gets soft, add in your chicken broth. Cover and cook for approximately 10 minutes.

9. Take out your chicken once it's done.

10. Add your lemon juice and cream. Allow it to simmer uncovered over a low heat for approximately 10 minutes. Mix a few times so your bottom doesn't burn.

11. Add in your mayo and mix. Turn off your burner.

12. Pull your chicken apart.

13. Add in half of your pulled chicken into cauliflower cream mix.

14. Use other 1/2 to line your 8x8-inch casserole dish.

15. On top of your bottom chicken layer, place your steamed chopped broccoli.

16. Top with your cauliflower cream mix.

17. Top that with your cheddar cheese.

18. Place in oven for approximately 30 minutes. Cover it with tinfoil.

19. Remove your tinfoil and cook for approximately 10 minutes.

20. Serve!

Bolognese Zoodle Bake (Serves 6)

Ingredients:

Bolognese Sauce:

1 1/2 pounds of Ground Beef

1/2 Medium White Onion

1 tablespoon of Olive Oil

2 cups of Rao's Marinara Sauce

3 cloves of Minced Garlic

1/2 teaspoon of Thyme

1/4 cup of Chicken Bouillon Paste

1/2 teaspoon of Ground Marjoram

1/2 teaspoon of Ground Nutmeg

2 tablespoons of Heavy Whipping Cream

Salt

Pepper

Zucchini Noodles:

3 Medium Zucchini

2 tablespoons of Olive Oil

1 cup of Shredded Mozzarella Cheese

Salt

Pepper

Fresh Basil (Optional)

Directions:

1. Preheat your skillet over a medium heat and set your slow cooker on "low." Finely dice half of your medium-sized white onion while you wait for your skillet to heat up.

2. Add your olive oil to your frying pan.

3. Once your oil becomes hot, add your diced onion. Cook until your onions start to become translucent and pick up a bit of color.

4. Stir in your minced garlic cloves.

5. Crumble your ground beef into the pan. Don't worry too much about breaking up the chunks as they cook. Everything is going to fall apart in the slow cooker anyway.

6. Add in 1/2 a teaspoon of thyme, 1/2 a teaspoon of nutmeg, 1/2 a teaspoon of marjoram, and black pepper.

7. Mix everything together and allow your beef to cook until it has mostly browned.

8. Mix in 2 cups of Rao's basil tomato marinara sauce.

9. Stir in 2 tablespoons of your heavy whipping cream.

10. Finish the sauce by mixing in 1/4 of a cup of your chicken bouillon.

11. Turn the heat off and allow the sauce to rest for approximately 10 minutes before transferring it into the preheated slow cooker. Be careful not to pour hot sauce into cold stoneware.

12. Cover your slow cooker and allow your sauce to simmer for about 8 hours. Stir occasionally to prevent burning. After the sauce has finished cooking you can season with additional salt if needed.

13. Preheat your oven to 350 degrees.

14. Set up a vegetable spiralizer. Use it to process the zucchini into noodles, and place the noodles in a casserole dish. Break apart the longer strands so that none of them are too long.

15. Add 2 tablespoons of olive oil to your noodles. Season to taste and then mix together.

16. Spread your Bolognese sauce over the top of your zucchini.

17. Top your casserole with 1 cup of shredded mozzarella cheese.

18. If baking right after cooking the Bolognese sauce, then you will only need to heat the casserole in the oven for approximately 15 to 20 minutes. If you've made the sauce ahead of time and it's been chilled in the refrigerator then you will need to bake for 30 to 35 minutes.

19. Garnish with fresh basil if desired.

20. Serve!

Nutritional Value:

402 Calories.

29 grams of Protein.

6 grams of Carbs.

29 grams of Fat.

Skillet Browned Chicken w/ Creamy Greens (Serves 4)

Ingredients:

1 pound of Boneless Chicken Thighs

1 cup of Chicken Stock

2 tablespoons of Coconut Oil

2 tablespoons of Melted Butter

1 cup of Cream

1 teaspoon of Italian Herbs

2 tablespoons of Coconut Flour

2 cups of Dark Leafy Greens

Pepper

Salt

Directions:

1. Preheat your large-sized skillet on a medium-high setting. Add 2 tablespoons of coconut oil to your pan. Season both sides of your chicken thighs with salt and pepper while your oil heats up. Brown your chicken thighs in the skillet.

2. Fry both sides until your chicken is cooked through and crispy. While your thighs are cooking you should start the sauce.

3. To create your sauce, melt 2 tablespoons of butter in your saucepan. Once your butter stops sizzling, whisk in 2 tablespoons of coconut flour to form a thick paste.

4. Whisk in 1 cup of cream and bring your mixture to a boil. The mixture should thicken after a few minutes. Stir in the teaspoon of Italian herbs.

5. Remove your cooked chicken thighs from the skillet and set to the side. Pour the cup of chicken stock into your chicken skillet and deglaze the pan. Whisk in your cream sauce. Stir the greens into your pan so that they become coated with your sauce.

6. Lay your chicken thighs back on top of the greens, then remove from the heat and serve. Divide your chicken and greens up into 4 servings.

7. Serve!

Nutritional Value:

446 Calories.

18 grams of Protein.

2 grams of Carbs.

38 grams of Fat.

Chicken Roulades w/ Sage & Gruyere (Serves 4)

Ingredients:

2 Chicken Breasts

1 Diced Medium Onion

1 tablespoon of Butter

3 ounces of Gruyere Cheese (Finely Grated)

1 tablespoon of White Wine Vinegar

2 tablespoons + 1 teaspoon of Chopped Fresh Sage

Salt

Pepper

Directions:

1. Preheat your oven to 375 degrees. Line an 11x13-inch baking pan with your parchment paper.

2. Butterfly each chicken breast. Place your knife along the side of the breast and use a sawing motion to carefully slice through the side, like opening a bagel. Be careful not to slice completely through the other side. Open the breast and lay flat.

3. Sandwich each of your chicken breasts between two pieces of plastic wrap. Using a meat tenderizing mallet, pound each breast until it is flat and about 1/4-inch thick. Sprinkle each side lightly with your salt and pepper.

4. Heat a medium-sized skillet over a medium heat. Add your butter.

5. When your butter stops foaming, add your onions to your skillet. Cook your onions over a medium-low heat until they caramelize, stirring frequently.

6. Add your white wine vinegar and stir, scraping up the browned bits. When the vinegar becomes syrupy, remove your pan from the heat. Add 2 tablespoons of sage and stir to combine. Season to taste with your salt and pepper.

7. Lay out three pieces of twine and place your flattened chicken breast on top.

8. Keeping the filling away from the edges, spread 1/2 of your onion sage mixture on each chicken breast. Sprinkle 2 ounces of grated cheese over each breast, reserving 1 ounce for later.

9. Roll each breast and secure tightly with twine or toothpicks.

10. Place in your baking pan and make sure they do not touch. Sprinkle your reserved cheese and sage over the roulades.

11. Bake in your preheated oven for approximately 35 minutes or until your chicken is cooked through. If the top is not sufficiently brown, place your chicken under the broiler for a few minutes at the end of cooking. Watch carefully as the cheese will brown quickly.

12. Remove from your oven and allow to cool for about 5 minutes before slicing. Remove your twine or toothpicks from the roulades. Carefully slice in a crosswise fashion.

13. Serve!

Nutritional Value:

315 Calories.

42 grams of Protein.

2 grams of Carbs.

14 grams of Fat.

BBQ Bacon Cheeseburger Waffles (Serves 4)

Ingredients:

Waffles:

1 1/2 ounces of Cheddar Cheese

3 tablespoons of Parmesan Cheese

2 Large Eggs

4 tablespoons of Almond Flour

1 cup of Cauliflower Crumbles

1/4 teaspoon of Onion Powder

1/4 teaspoon of Garlic Powder

Salt

Pepper

Topping:

4 ounces of Ground Beef (70/30)

4 slices of Chopped Bacon

4 tablespoons of Sugar-Free BBQ Sauce

1 1/2 ounces of Cheddar Cheese

Salt

Pepper

Directions:

1. Shred up 3 ounces worth of cheese. Half will go into your waffle and half will go on top, so make sure you keep it to the side.

2. Mix in half of your cheddar cheese, Parmesan cheese, eggs, almond flour, and spices. Set to the side.

3. Slice your bacon thin and cook over a medium-high heat.

4. Once your bacon is partially cooked, add in your beef.

5. Add any excess grease from your pan into your waffle mixture that you have set to the side.

6. Immersion blend your waffle mixture into a thick paste.

7. Add half of your mixture to your waffle iron and cook until it's crisp. Keep in mind that cauliflower waffles tend to take a little bit longer to cook (there's much more moisture). A good rule of thumb to use is that the waffle is finished once there is little to no steam coming from the waffle iron. Repeat for the second waffle.

8. While your waffles are cooking, add in your sugar-free BBQ sauce to the bacon and ground beef mixture in your pan.

9. Assemble your waffles together by adding half of the ground beef mixture and half of the remaining cheddar cheese to the top of your waffle.

10. Broil for 1 to 2 minutes or until your cheese is nicely melted over the top.

11. Slice up your green onion while your pizzas are broiling to sprinkle over the top.

12. Serve!

Nutritional Value:

354 Calories.

19 grams of Protein.

3 grams of Carbs.

30 grams of Fat.

Chicken Thighs w/ Spinach (Serves 8)

Ingredients:

16 Boneless Chicken Thighs (Skinless)

2 tablespoons of Shredded Cheddar Cheese

24 ounces of Spinach

2 cups of Water

Garlic

Salt

Pepper

Directions:

1. Place your chicken thighs into your roaster pan covered with your lid.

2. Bake at 350 degrees for approximately 2 hours.

3. Remove and allow it to cool.

4. Place 2 thighs each in 8 different containers.

5. Break up your thighs and place your vegetables and cheese on each.

6. Distribute your leftover juices over the chicken in each container.

7. Serve!

Nutritional Value:

390 Calories.

45 grams of Protein.

3 grams of Carbs.

23 grams of Fat.

Loaded Baked Chicken (Serves 4)

Ingredients:

4 Chicken Breasts

4 Bacon Strips

1 ounce of Soy Sauce

4 ounces of Cheddar Cheese

4 ounces of Ranch Dressing

3 Green Onions

Directions:

1. Heat your cast iron pan and cook your oil on a high heat.

2. Pan fry your chicken breasts. Flip them half way through. Total cook time should be approximately 10 to 15 minutes. Internal temperature should be 165 degrees.

3. While your chicken cooks, cook your bacon and crumble into bits when done.

4. Chop up your green onions.

5. Place your chicken in your baking dish. Top it with your soy sauce, then add your ranch, bacon, green onions, and your cheese.

6. Broil on high for approximately 3 to 4 minutes until your cheese melts.

7. Serve!

Nutritional Value:

527 Calories.

63 grams of Protein.

3 grams of Carbs.

28 grams of Fat.

Beer Can Chicken (Serves 4)

Ingredients:

1 Whole Chicken

1 tablespoon of Bacon Fat

1 can of Beer

Rotisserie Seasoning

Directions:

1. Preheat your grill to a medium-high heat, Set it up for indirect grilling. No heat under the chicken.

2. Remove and get rid of your gizzards from your thawed chicken.

3. Cut away the loose skin and chicken parts from the opening of breast cavity.

4. Dry it on both the outside and inside.

5. Apply oil or bacon fat to the outside of your chicken.

6. Rub in your Rotisserie seasoning on both inside and outside.

7. Remove half of the beer from the can and set your chicken on the can.

8. Grill for approximately 60 minutes or until your meat reads between 165 and 180 degrees.

9. Allow it to rest for 5 to 10 minutes.

10. Serve!

Garlic Lebanese Chicken Thighs (Serves 2)

Ingredients:

4 Chicken Thighs

1 Vidalia Onion (Quartered)

2 Roma Tomatoes

2 tablespoons of Ghee

15 whole cloves of Garlic

1 Juiced Fresh Lemon

Handful of Baby Carrots

Garlic Olive Oil

Oregano

Pepper

Salt

Directions:

1. Heat your oven to 500 degrees.

2. Glaze the bottom of your cast iron pan with 2 teaspoons of garlic olive oil.

3. Add your 4 chicken thighs together. Make sure some space separate them.

4. Wedge your carrots, onions, tomatoes, and garlic cloves between your chicken thighs. Add 2 garlic cloves on top of the thighs.

5. Juice your lemon over your chicken thighs.

6. Drizzle more garlic oil over the top of your chicken thighs.

7. Drizzle ghee over your chicken thighs.

8. Sprinkle your oregano over your dish. Add your pepper and salt.

9. Place in oven for approximately 30 minutes.

10. Reduce your heat to 350 degrees and then cook approximately 20 minutes until cooked to an internal temperature of 165 degrees.

11. Place your oven on broil and cook an additional 5 minutes until outside the skin is crispy.

12. Remove from your oven.

13. Serve!

Tequila Chicken (Serves 6)

Ingredients:

Marinade:

6 Chicken Breasts

1/2 teaspoon of Garlic Powder

1 cup of Water

1/2 teaspoon of Liquid Smoke

1/4 cup of Soy Sauce

2 tablespoons of Lime Juice

1 shot of Tequila (50 ml)

1/2 teaspoon of Salt

Sauce:

1/4 cup of Sour Cream

1/4 cup of Tomato Sauce

1/4 cup of Mayonnaise

1/4 teaspoon of Frank's Hot Sauce

1 tablespoon of Heavy Cream

1/4 teaspoon of Dried Dill

1/4 teaspoon of Cayenne Pepper

1/4 teaspoon of Dried Parsley

6 ounces of Shredded Cheddar Cheese

1/4 teaspoon of Paprika

1/4 teaspoon of Chili Powder

1/4 teaspoon of Ground Cumin

1/4 teaspoon of Salt

1/4 teaspoon of Black Pepper

Directions:

1. Mix together your marinade ingredients.

2. Add your chicken to the marinade. Allow it to sit and refrigerate for approximately 2 to 3 hours.

3. Place your chicken on your broiler pan and then broil for approximately 20 minutes on high. Flip it after 10 minutes.

4. Check chicken for temperature. You want it to get to 165 degrees internally.

5. Mix all your ingredients for your sauce except the cheese.

6. Place your meat in your casserole dish. Cover it with sauce and your cheese.

7. Broil for 3 more minutes on high. Cheese should be a little bubbly.

8. Serve!

Nutritional Value:

445 Calories.

60 grams of Protein.

2 grams of Carbs.

22 grams of Fat.

Pounded Chicken Pizza (Serves 4)

Ingredients:

4 Chicken Thighs

16 slices of Pepperoni

2 1/2 ounces of Shredded Jarlsberg Cheese

4 slices of Bacon

2 1/2 ounces of Shredded Cheddar Cheese

1/2 cup of Marinara Sauce

1 ounce of Shredded Monterey Cheese

Italian Seasoning

Pepper

Salt

Directions:

1. Preheat your oven to 350 degrees.

2. Start cooking your 4 slices of bacon.

3. Place your chicken thighs on cutting board. Cover it with saran wrap. Pound it with your heavy pan.

4. Pepper and salt both sides of your chicken.

5. Heat up grease in your pan over a high heat. Sear your chicken on each side for 1 minute.

6. Transfer your skillet to your oven and cook for approximately 10 minutes.

7. Remove your skillet from the oven. Add your seasoning and sauce.

8. Cover it with cheese and place back in your oven for approximately 3 minutes on broil.

9. Remove from oven. Add your remaining toppings. This includes pepperoni and bacon. Broil for 2 more minutes.

10. Serve!

Nutritional Value:

461 Calories.

32 grams of Protein.

1 gram of Carbs.

36 grams of Fat.

Beer Can Burgers (Serves 5)

Ingredients:

50 ounces of Ground Beef

2 1/2 ounces of Pepper Jack Cheese (Cubed)

10 slices of Bacon

2 1/2 ounces of Shredded Extra Sharp Cheddar Cheese

6 ounces of Cooked Sliced Fresh Mushrooms

6 ounces of Cooked Brussels Sprouts

6 ounces of Cooked Green Peppers

6 ounces of Cooked Onions

Directions:

1. Preheat your grill to 300 degrees. Set it up for indirect heat.

2. Divide your ground beef into equal amounts and make them into large balls.

3. Push a can into your ball and smush it.

4. Using your own hand, form the meat around your can, making sure to push it up evenly around your can.

5. Wrap 2 pieces of bacon around the base of your meat.

6. Extract your can and fill the hole with whatever you'd like. In this example, we used green peppers, onions, brussels sprouts, and mushrooms.

7. Top it with your cheese.

8. Place on your grill and cook with indirect heat for approximately 1 hour.

9. Take off your grill.

10. Serve!

<u>Nutritional Value:</u>

963 Calories.

66 grams of Protein.

8 grams of Carbs.

73 grams of Fat.

Juicy Sliders (Serves 4)

Ingredients:

1 Egg

8 ounces of Cheddar Cheese

1 pound of Ground Beef

Dash of Worcestershire Sauce

Onion Powder

Garlic

Salt

Pepper

Directions:

1. Mix your eggs, spices, and beef.

2. Divide your meat into patties of 1 1/2 ounces.

3. Add a 1/2 ounce of cheese to each of your patties.

4. Combine two of your patties to form one burger. Use your hands to meld the two patties together.

5. Heat oil on high and then fry your burgers to your desired level.

6. Top with your cheese and your desired toppings.

7. Serve!

Nutritional Value:

285 Calories.

22 grams of Protein.

0 grams of Carbs.

21 grams of Fat.

Bacon Wrapped Brats (Serves 4)

Ingredients:

4 Bacon Slices

2 12-ounce Beers

4 slices of Cheese

4 Brats

4 Romaine Lettuce Leafs

Directions:

1. Place your brats in your pot. Cover it with your beer.

2. Boil for approximately 10 minutes.

3. Remove your brats and wrap them with your bacon.

4. Grill your bacon wrapped brats until your bacon gets crisp.

5. Serve!

Flank Steak Pinwheels (Serves 6)

Ingredients:

2 pounds of Flank Steak

16 ounces of Mozzarella Cheese

8 ounces of Fresh Spinach

Italian Seasoning

Directions:

1. Preheat your oven to 350 degrees.

2.Place your flank steak so your grain is going right to left.

3. Square your flank and remove the hard fat deposits.

4. Using a sharp knife, butterfly your steak. Be sure to cut parallel to your cutting board leaving about an inch not cut. Always cut along the grain.

5. Open your steak, using your knife to finish off the cut so a 1/2 is still connected.

6. Lay your steak flat. Grain needs to be facing up and down your cutting board.

7. Season each side with Italian seasoning.

8. Spread your mozzarella cheese over your steak. Leave an inch on one of your sides for wrapping.

9. Lay down 2 layers of spinach.

10. Roll your steak. Be sure to keep it tight, rolling it with your grain.

11. Cut 6 pieces of twine and then tie off 6 sections spaced evenly.

12. Cut out your pinwheels carefully by cutting between twine pieces.

13. Place in your Pyrex baking dish over a layer of spinach.

14. Cook for approximately 25 minutes.

15. Broil for about 3 minutes until your cheese is bubbly.

16. Serve!

Nutritional Value:

519 Calories.

57 grams of Protein.

1 gram of Carbs.

29 grams of Fat.

Fat Burning Ginger Steak (Serves 2)

Ingredients:

2 Sirloin Steaks (Each 4 Ounces)

4 tablespoons of Apple Cider Vinegar

1 Diced Small Onion

2 Small Diced Tomatoes

1 clove of Crushed Garlic

1 tablespoon of Olive Oil

1 teaspoon of Ground Ginger

Pepper

Salt

Directions:

1. Place your oil in your large-sized skillet. Brown your steaks over a medium-high heat.

2. Once each side is seared, add in your tomatoes, garlic, and onion.

3. In your bowl, add your salt, pepper, and ginger into your vinegar and then add your mixture to your skillet. Stir together well to combine.

4. Cover your skillet. Turn your heat to low and allow it to simmer until your liquids are completely evaporated.

5. Serve!

Nutritional Value:

208 Calories.

31 grams of Protein.

3 grams of Carbs.

8 grams of Fat.

Stuffed & Seared Flank Steak (Serves 6)

Ingredients:

2 Flank Steaks

16 ounces of Spinach

7 ounces of Roasted Red Peppers

1 Egg Yolk

4 ounces of Bleu Cheese

2 tablespoons of Almond Flour

1/2 teaspoon of Garlic Powder

1/2 teaspoon of Onion Powder

1/2 teaspoon of Pepper

1/2 teaspoon of Salt

Directions:

1. Place the grain of your flank steak vertically.

2. Butterfly your steak cutting from right to left.

3. Microwave your frozen spinach and then drain any liquid.

4. Slice your roasted red peppers.

5. Combine your remaining ingredients with your spinach. Mix together well.

6. Spread your mixture over your steak and then roll with your grain.

7. Truss your steak with some cotton twine.

8. Wrap it with saran wrap. Marinate it for approximately 30 minutes.

9. Cook for approximately 35 minutes at 425 degrees.

10. Broil steak for around 10 minutes. Rotate steak after approximately 5 minutes.

11. Cover it with your foil. Rest for approximately 10 minutes.

12. Serve!

Nutritional Value:

470 Calories.

54 grams of Protein.

6 grams of Carbs.

25 grams of Fat.

Bacon Wrapped Filet Mignon w/ Bleu Cheese Butter (Serves 8)

Ingredients:

Bacon Wrapped Filet Mignon:

8 Filet Mignon Steaks. (10 Ounces Each / 3-Inch Thick Cut)

8 slices of Bacon

Salt

Pepper

Bleu Cheese Butter:

2 tablespoons of Minced Garlic

1/4 teaspoon of Montreal Steak Seasoning

Stick of Butter

1/4 teaspoon of Dried Thyme

1/4 teaspoon of Onion Powder

Directions:

Bleu Cheese Butter:

1. Soften your butter. Once soft add to your food processor.

2. Add the rest of your bleu cheese butter ingredients except bleu cheese.

3. Mince your mixture until it is blended.

4. Add your bleu cheese and mix together well.

5. Transfer to your container and refrigerate.

Bacon Wrapped Filet Mignon:

6. Bring your meat to room temperature. Should take approximately 30 minutes.

7. Pepper and salt both sides.

8. Wrap your bacon and secure it with a toothpick.

9. Sear it on high heat. Do so in an oven proof skillet. Sear for approximately 3 minutes on both sides.

10. Transfer to your oven and set at 450 degrees.

11. Should take approximately 8 to 10 minutes to cook for each steak. Check your meat for desired preference.

12. Add you your bleu cheese butter to your steaks as desired.

13. Serve!

Nutritional Value:

598 Calories.

61 grams of Protein.

1 grams of Carbs.

37 grams of Fat.

Steak w/ Mushroom Port Sauce (Serves 2)

Ingredients:

2 pounds of Rib Eye Steak

10 ounces of Mushrooms

2 ounces of Heavy Cream

4 ounces of Port Wine

1 tablespoon of Butter

Salt

Pepper

Directions:

1. Preheat your oven to 450 degrees.

2. Pepper and salt each side of your steak.

3. Heat your cast iron skillet on a high heat.

4. Melt your butter until it bubbles.

5. Cook your steak for approximately 2 minutes on each side and then move to your oven for finishing.

6. Cook in your oven until the internal temperature is above 135 degrees. The higher the temp the more well done it will be. Should take about 12 minutes. Be sure to flip steaks at the 6-minute mark.

7. Once your steaks are finished remove them from the oven and cover with some foil.

8. Add your port wine to your pan to deglaze. Scrap the bits of burnt stuff from the bottom.

9. Add your cream and mushrooms. Light on fire.

10. Once your sauce has gotten thicker, pour it over your steak.

11. Serve!

Nutritional Value:

984 Calories.

102 grams of Protein.

6 grams of Carbs.

62 grams of Fat.

Parmesan Encrusted Pork Chops (Serves 14)

Ingredients:

14 Bone-In Pork Chops

6 ounces of Parmesan Cheese

2 Large Eggs

3/4 cup of Almond Flour

Salt

Pepper

Directions:

1. Grate your Parmesan cheese and combine it with your almond flour and spices.

2. Whisk your eggs and put in your shallow container.

3. Dip your pork chops in your eggs and coat with your Parmesan mix.

4. Fry your pork chops in your bacon grease in your pan for approximately 1 minute on each side.

5. Cook at 400 degrees in your oven for approximately 10 minutes or until it is done to the desired preference. The amount of time will depend on the thickness of your pork chops.

6. Serve!

Nutritional Value:

454 Calories.

33 grams of Protein.

4 grams of Carbs.

34 grams of Fat.

Pan Fried Pork Chops (Serves 3)

Ingredients:

3 Bone-In Pork Chops

1 tablespoon of Butter

1/2 cup of Coconut Flour

1/4 teaspoon of Cayenne Pepper

1 teaspoon of Black Pepper

1 teaspoon of Seasoned Salt

Directions:

1. Mix all your dry ingredients together in a container big enough to fit your pork chops.

2. Dry your pork chops.

3. Heat your skillet on high. Add in your butter.

4. Coat your pork chops in the dry mix and fry.

5. Cook for approximately 5 minutes per side until it is done to your preference.

6. Serve!

Nutritional Value:

298 Calories.

27 grams of Protein.

11 grams of Carbs.

15 grams of Fat.

Keto Asian Pork Chops (Serves 2)

Ingredients:

4 Boneless Pork Chops

1 Medium Star Anise

1 stalk of Lemon Grass (Diced & Peeled)

4 halved Garlic Cloves

1 tablespoon of Almond Flour

1/2 tablespoon of Sugar-Free Ketchup

1 tablespoon of Fish Sauce

1/2 tablespoon of Sambal Chili Paste

1/2 teaspoon of Five Spice

1 1/2 teaspoons of Soy Sauce

1/2 teaspoon of Peppercorns

1 teaspoon of Sesame Oil

Directions:

1. Place your pork chops on a flat surface and use your rolling pin wrapped in some wax paper to pound your chops to 1/2-inch thickness.

2. Cut your garlic cloves in half.

3. Grind your star anise and peppercorns to a fine powder using your blender. Add your garlic and lemon grass. Blend until in puree form. Add your soy sauce, fish sauce, five-spice, and sesame oil. Mix it together well.

4. Place your pork chops on a tray and pour on your marinade. Coat on both sides. Cover and allow it to marinate at room temperature for approximately 2 hours.

5. Sear your pork chops on both sides in your pan. Should take approximately 2 minutes on both sides. Should see a golden brown crust forming.

6. Transfer over to your cutting board and cut each of your chops into strips.

7. To make your sauce, stir your Sambal chili paste and ketchup together.

8. Serve!

Nutritional Values:

272 Calories.

34 grams of Protein.

6 grams of Carbs.

9.5 grams of Fat.

Blackened Pork Chops (Serves 4)

Ingredients:

4 Pork Chops

1 teaspoon of Onion Powder

1 tablespoon of Paprika

1/2 teaspoon of Oregano Leaves

1 teaspoon of Garlic Powder

4 tablespoons of Butter

1/4 teaspoon of Cayenne Pepper

1/2 teaspoon of Thyme Leaves

1 teaspoon of Cumin

2 teaspoons of Salt

2 teaspoons of Black Pepper

Directions:

1. Assemble your spices and mix it in your shallow-sized bowl big enough to fit your pork chop.

2. Melt your butter in a different bowl.

3. Heat up some bacon grease in your skillet.

4. Dip your chops in butter and coat with your spices. Put it in your oil.

5. Cook for approximately 3 to 5 minutes per side.

6. Flip once and cook until your temperature reaches between 140 to 150 degrees.

7. Serve!

Nutritional Value:

341 Calories.

46 grams of Protein.

4 grams of Carbs.

15 grams of Fat.

Reuben Casserole (Serves 4)

Ingredients:

12 ounces of Cooked Corned Beef

8 ounces of Jarlsberg

1 Small Onion

4 ounces of Cheddar Cheese

1 can of Sauerkraut

1/2 cup of Thousand Island Dressing

1/4 cup of Mayo

Pepper

Directions:

1. Slice and dice your corned beef. Add it to your large-sized bowl.

2. Use a grater with a large opening, shred your onion, add it to your bowl.

3. Use the same grater on your Jarlsberg, add it to your bowl.

4. Drain your can of Sauerkraut, add it to your bowl.

5. Add your cheddar cheese to your bowl.

6. Add your mayo and Thousand Island dressing to your bowl.

7. Add some fresh pepper.

8. Mix together and spread into your 8-inch greased pan.

9. Cook for approximately 35 minutes at 350 degrees.

10. Serve!

Nutritional Value:

769 Calories.

37 grams of Protein.

10 grams of Carbs.

63 grams of Fat.

Crockpot Corned Beef & Cabbage (Serves 10)

Ingredients:

6 pounds of Corned Beef

1 Small Onion

4 cups of Water

4 Carrots

1 Celery Bunch

1/2 teaspoon of Ground Coriander

1/2 teaspoon of Ground Mustard

1 Large Cabbage Head

1/2 teaspoon of Ground Thyme

1/2 teaspoon of Allspice

1/2 teaspoon of Ground Marjoram

1/2 teaspoon of Salt

1/2 teaspoon of Black Pepper

Directions:

1. Cut up your celery, carrots, and onions.

2. Line your crockpot with your vegetables.

3. Add your water.

4. Mix your spices all together.

5. Rub each side of your corned beef with your spices and put on top of your vegetables.

6. Cover and then cook in your crockpot on low for approximately 7 hours.

7. Discard the top layer of your cabbage. Wash and then quarter.

8. Put your cabbage in your crockpot. Cook for another hour on low.

9. Serve!

Nutritional Value:

583 Calories.

42 grams of Protein.

13 grams of Carbs.

40 grams of Fat.

Kimchi Shirataki Noodles (Serves 4)

Ingredients:

2 House Foods Tofu Shirataki Noodles

4 ounces of Sliced Pork Belly

1/2 container of Kimchi

1 tablespoon of Sesame Oil

1 tablespoon of Soy Sauce

1 tablespoon of Fish Sauce

4 stalks of Green Onions

Directions:

1. Prep your ingredients.

2. Cut your pork belly into small pieces.

3. Cut your kimchi into smaller bite size pieces.

4. Wash your noodles.

5. Add your oils to your wok and heat it on high.

6. Add your pork belly and fry it for a few minutes until it's cooked.

7. Throw in your kimchi and continue to fry it.

8. Make a hole in the middle of your wok. Add your noodles. Fry until hot.

9. Transfer to your bowl and top it with your green onions.

10. Serve!

Nutritional Value:

221 Calories.

6 grams of Protein.

6 grams of Carbs.

19 grams of Fat.

Mahi-Mahi w/ Hummus (Serves 1)

Ingredients:

1 Mahi Mahi Filet

1 teaspoon of Philadelphia Cheese

1 cup of Frozen Vegetables

1 tablespoon of Lime

2 tablespoons of Hummus

Fresh Coriander

Cilantro

Sea Salt

Ground Pepper

Directions:

1. Place your vegetables on the bottom steamer basket and your Mahi Mahi on the top steamer basket.

2. Add your lime, pepper, salt, and cilantro.

3. Set your steamer for approximately 30 minutes.

4. Add cheese on your vegetables and your hummus as a side dish.

5. Serve!

Nutritional Value:

228 Calories.

35 grams of Protein.

10 grams of Carbs.

7 grams of Fat.

.

Coconut Shrimp & Avocado (Serves 1)

Ingredients:

1 cup of Shrimp

1/2 Avocado

1/2 tablespoon of Organic Peanut Butter

1 teaspoon of Shredded Coconut

1 tablespoon of Light Coconut Milk

Olive Oil

Sriracha Hot Sauce

Directions:

1. Set your nonstick saute pan over a medium heat. Spray with your olive oil.

2. Pour in your Sriracha, coconut milk, and peanut butter.

3. Add your shrimp and saute for approximately 3 to 4 minutes until your shrimps turn pink.

4. Cut your half of an avocado into cubes and place on your plate.

5. Add your shrimps on top of your avocado and sprinkle with your shredded coconut.

6. Serve!

Nutritional Value:

250 Calories.

24 grams of Protein.

11 grams of Carbs.

12 grams of Fat.

Keto Baked Salmon

Ingredients:

2 pounds of Salmon Fillets

4 ounces of Sesame Oil

1/2 cup of Tamari Soy Sauce

1/2 teaspoon of Ground Ginger

1 teaspoon of Minced Garlic

1/2 teaspoon of Rosemary

1/4 teaspoon of Tarragon

1/4 teaspoon of Thyme

1 teaspoon of Oregano Leaves

1/2 teaspoon of Basil

1/2 teaspoon of Rosemary

1/2 cup of Chopped Green Onions

4 ounces of Butter

1/2 cup of Chopped Fresh Mushrooms

Directions:

1. Cut your fillet into 1/2 pound pieces. Get out a 1-quart freezer Ziploc bag.

2. Stir together your spices, sesame oil, and tamari sauce. Put your salmon in your Ziploc bag and then pour in your sauce mix.

3. Refrigerate your salmon with the skin side facing up in your marinade for approximately 1 to 4 hours.

4. Preheat your oven to 350 degrees. Line your large-sized baking pan with foil.

5. Pour out your fillets and marinade into your pan. Lay out your fish in a single layer.

6. Bake your fillets for approximately 10 to 15 minutes.

7. While your salmon cooks prepare your vegetables.

8. Melt your butter. Add your vegetables to it and mix to coat your vegetables.

9. Remove your salmon from the oven and pour your butter mixture over your salmon so each one is covered.

10. Bake for approximately 10 more minutes at 350 degrees.

11. Serve!

Nutritional Value:

353 Calories.

32 grams of Protein.

2 grams of Carbs.

23 grams of Fat.

Keto Meatloaf (Serves 12)

Ingredients:

2 pounds of 85% Ground Beef

1 pound of Italian Sausage

8 ounces of Chopped White Onion

2 Large Eggs

2 tablespoons of Butter

1/2 cup of Almond Flour

5 Minced Garlic Cloves

1/2 cup of Dry Grated Parmesan Cheese

1 cup of Chopped Green Pepper

1 tablespoon of Thyme Leaves

1/4 cup of Minced Fresh Parsley Leaves

1 tablespoon of Chopped Fresh Basil Leaves

1/4 cup of Heavy Cream

2 tablespoons of Ellen's Low-Carb BBQ Sauce

2 teaspoons of Dijon Mustard

1/2 teaspoon of Unflavored Gelatin

1/2 teaspoon of Ground Black Pepper

1 teaspoon of Salt

Directions:

1. Preheat your oven to 350 degrees. Grease your 10x15-inch baking dish with your butter. Place to the side.

2. In your small-sized deep bowl, whisk your Parmesan cheese and almond flour together. Place to the side.

3. Heat your butter in your medium-sized skillet over a medium heat. Add your garlic, pepper, and onion. Saute until softened. Should be approximately 8 minutes. Place to the side to cool while getting your other ingredients ready. Once your mixture is cool, run it through your food processor to mince your vegetables to a fine consistency.

4. In a separate deep small-sized bowl, whisk your pepper, salt, spices, eggs, BBQ sauce, cream, and mustard. Sprinkle your gelatin over the mixture. Allow it to stand for approximately 5 minutes. Add in your minced onion mixture and mix together well. Place to the side.

5. Place your ground beef and sausage on your large-sized cutting board, Mix them together. Make sure no large chunks are left unmixed. Don't knead your meat for more than 5 minutes. If you do it will make your meat tough.

6. Return your low-carb meatloaf to a large-sized mixing bowl. Add in your egg mix and mix together well. Add in your almond flour mixture. Mix until it is evenly blended together. It should no longer be sticky.

7. Place in your baking dish, making it into a loaf. Leave approximately an inch on all sides. Flatten your loaf shape on top so it all will cook evenly.

8. Bake your meatloaf until it is browned. Your cooking thermometer should read at least 160 degrees. It should take approximately 1 hour. Allow it to rest for approximately 20 minutes.

9. Serve!

Nutritional Value:

409 Calories.

23 grams of Protein.

5 grams of Carbs.

33 grams of Fat.

Chapter Four: Ketogenic Diet Snacks, Drinks, & Condiment Recipes

In this section, I will give you 30+ keto snacks, drinks, & condiment recipes you can make yourself. I'll include both basic recipes and a few more advanced recipes. That way no matter what your level is in the kitchen you'll be able to prepare yourself a healthy low-carb ketogenic snack, drink, or condiment to keep you on track with your diet. I'll add in the nutritional value whenever possible, although I don't always have those exact numbers for each and every recipe.

Keto 5 Layer Dip (Serves 10)

Ingredients:

20 ounces of Guacamole

4 ounces of Diced Green Onions

8 ounces of Sour Cream

4 ounces of Mayo

16 ounces of Salsa

4 ounces of Cream Cheese

10 ounces of Shredded Cheddar Cheese

2 tablespoons of Taco Seasoning

Directions:

1. Combine your mayo, cream cheese, sour cream, and seasoning.

2. Mix until smooth.

3. Chop your green onions.

4. Layer 1 - Use your medium-sized casserole dish and spread out your guacamole on the bottom.

5. Layer 2 - Carefully spread your sour cream mix over top your guacamole.

6. Layer 3 - Spread your salsa over your sour cream mixture.

7. Layer 4 - Add your cheese.

8. Layer 5 - Top with your green onions.

9. Refrigerate it least 1 hour.

10. Serve!

Nutritional Value:

343 Calories.

10 grams of Protein.

11 grams of Carbs.

29 grams of Fat.

Spicy Bacon Cauliflower (Serves 4)

Ingredients:

16 ounces of Frozen Cauliflower

5 slices of Thick Cut Bacon

Old Bay

Directions:

1. Microwave your entire bag of cauliflower.

2. Cook your bacon until it is crisp in your oven at 450 degrees.

3. Heat your bacon grease in your skillet.

4. Add your cooked cauliflower to your grease and cover heavily with your Old Bay.

5. Saute this for approximately 5 minutes. Be sure to mix around well.

6. Reapply your Old Bay.

7. Mix until your cauliflower is well cooked and broken up.

8. Take your bacon out of your oven and cut into small pieces. Add it to your mixture.

9. Serve!

Nutritional Value:

100 Calories.

6 grams of Protein.

5 grams of Carbs.

6 grams of Fat.

Cheesy Cauliflower Onion Dip (Serves 24)

Ingredients:

1 pound of Cauliflower

1/2 cup of Onion

1 1/2 cups of Chicken Broth

3/4 cup of Cream Cheese

1/4 cup of Mayonnaise

1/2 teaspoon of Ground Cumin

1/2 teaspoon of Garlic Powder

1/2 teaspoon of Chili Powder

1/2 teaspoon of Ground Black Pepper

1/2 teaspoon of Salt

Directions:

1. Simmer your cauliflower and onion in your chicken broth until soft and tender.

2. Stir in your garlic powder, cumin, chili powder, pepper, and salt.

3. Cut up chunks of your cream cheese and whisk into your cauliflower until the cream cheese melts and is no longer chunky.

4. Use a blender to blend your mixture until it's smooth.

5. Carefully whisk in your mayonnaise.

6. Chill in your fridge for approximately 2 to 3 hours.

7. Serve!

Nutritional Value:

51 Calories.

1 grams of Protein.

1 grams of Carbs.

4 grams of Fat.

Pesto Keto Crackers (Serves 6)

Ingredients:

1 1/4 cups of Almond Flour

1/4 teaspoon of Dried Basil

1/2 teaspoon of Baking Powder

1 clove of Pressed Garlic

3 tablespoons of Butter

2 tablespoons of Basil Pesto

Pinch of Cayenne Pepper

1/4 teaspoon of Ground Black Pepper

1/2 teaspoon of Salt

Directions:

1. Preheat your oven to 325 degrees. Line your cookie sheet with parchment paper.

2. In your medium-sized bowl, combine your almond flour, pepper, salt and baking powder and whisk until smooth.

3. Add your basil, cayenne, and garlic and stir until evenly combined.

4. Add in your pesto and whisk until your dough forms into coarse crumbs.

5. Cut the butter into your cracker mixture with a fork or your fingers until your dough forms into a ball.

6. Transfer your dough onto the prepared cookie sheet and spread out your dough thinly until it's about 1 1/2 mm thick. Make sure the thickness is the same throughout so that the crackers bake evenly.

7. Place your pan in the preheated oven and bake for approximately 14 to 17 minutes until light golden brown in color.

8. Once your dough has finished baking, remove it from the oven.

9. Cut into crackers of your desired size or allow it to cool and then break it into pieces.

10. Serve!

Nutritional Value:

210 Calories.

5 grams of Protein.

3 grams of Carbs.

20 grams of Fat.

Mini Pumpkin Spice Muffins (Serves 18)

Ingredients:

3/4 cup of Canned Pumpkin

1 Large Egg (Room Temperature)

1/4 cup of Organic No Sugar Added Sunflower Seed Butter

1/2 teaspoon of Ground Nutmeg

1/2 cup of Erythritol

2 tablespoons of Organic Flaxseed Meal

1/4 cup of Organic Coconut Flour (Sifted)

1/2 teaspoon of Baking Powder

1 teaspoon of Ground Cinnamon

1/2 teaspoon of Baking Soda

1/4 teaspoon of Salt

3 tablespoons of Plain Cream Cheese (Optional)

Directions:

1. Preheat your oven to 350 degrees then lightly grease your mini muffin pan. You will need 18 sections to bake your entire recipe. Then in your mixing bowl combine your pumpkin, sunflower seed butter, and your egg. Stir until smooth.

2. Add all of your remaining dry ingredients.

3. Stir to blend.

4. Using a 1-tablespoon measuring spoon, scoop your batter into your prepared pan. Bake approximately 15 minutes, then remove your pan from the oven and allow it to cool completely.

5. Carefully remove your muffins from your pan and transfer to your serving tray. You can optionally top your muffins with cream cheese.

6. Store in a sealed container at room temperature for up to 3 days. You may also refrigerate your muffins up to 1 week, or freeze up to 1 month. They are best when warmed slightly if refrigerated or frozen. If freezing, do not top with cream cheese until thawed.

7. Serve!

Nutritional Value:

43 Calories.

2 grams of Protein.

2.5 grams of Carbs.

3 grams of Fat.

Keto Tortilla Chips (Serves 36)

Ingredients:

Tortilla Chips:

6 Tortillas

3 tablespoons of Oil

Pepper

Salt

Optional Toppings:

Diced Jalapeno

Shredded Cheese

Fresh Salsa

Full-Fat Sour Cream

Directions:

1. Cut your tortillas into chip-sized slices. I got 6 out of each tortilla.

2. Heat your deep fryer. Once ready, lay out the pieces of your tortilla in your basket. You can fry 4 to 6 pieces at a time.

3. Fry for about 1 to 2 minutes, then flip. Continue to fry for another 1 to 2 minutes on the other side.

4. Remove from your fryer and place on paper towels to cool. Season with your salt and pepper to taste.

5. Add your toppings of choice.

6. Serve!

Nutritional Value:

27 Calories.

1 gram of Protein.

.04 grams of Carbs.

3 grams of Fat.

Bacon Brussels Sprouts (Serves 4)

Ingredients:

1/4 cup of Fish Sauce

6 strips of Bacon

1/4 cup of Bacon Grease or Oil

24 ounces of Brussels Sprouts

Pepper

Directions:

1. De-stem and quarter your brussels sprouts.

2. Mix your brussels sprouts, fish sauce, and bacon grease.

3. Cook your bacon. Once done cut into smaller strips.

4. Add your bacon to your mix and add some pepper. Stir together well.

5. On your greased pan spread out your brussels sprouts.

6. Cook for approximately 40 minutes at 450 degrees, stirring in 10-minute intervals.

7. Finish off your brussels sprouts on broil for a couple of minutes.

8. Serve!

Nutritional Value:

143 Calories.

6 grams of Protein.

8 grams of Carbs.

10 grams of Fat.

Kohlrabi Kraut (Serves 12)

Ingredients:

2 pounds of Ham Hock

12 ounces of Salt Pork

4 Shredded Kohlrabi

1/2 of an Onion

1/2 cup of Champagne Vinegar

1 teaspoon of Caraway Seeds

Directions:

1. Fill your large-sized pot halfway with water and boil on a high heat.

2. Add your bacon grease to your skillet and heat on high.

3. Cut up 1/4 of an onion.

4. Brown your ham hocks in bacon grease.

5. Add your onions to your pan and fry with your ham hocks.

6. Once your onions get cooked and ham hocks are browned, add to boiling water and season with your pepper and salt.

7. Peel and quarter your kohlrabi.

8. Grate your kohlrabi in your food processor.

9. Grate 1/4 of an onion into your mix.

10. Add your kohlrabi to water and season it with your pepper and salt.

11. Add your caraway seeds and champagne vinegar.

12. Cover and allow it to simmer approximately 3 hours. Stir occasionally.

13. If water gets low while simmering add more. The mixture should be covered with water for entire 3 hours.

14. Near the end of simmer remove ham hocks and separate the bone from the meat. Add your meat back into your pot.

15. Serve!

Nutritional Value:

181 Calories.

14 grams of Protein.

7 grams of Carbs.

17 grams of Fat.

Bacon Rollups (Serves 1)

Ingredients:

2 slices of Bacon

2 slices of Cheddar Cheese

2 Toothpicks

Directions:

1. Cut each cheese piece vertically into fours.

2. Cook your bacon until it is crisp.

3 Remove your bacon and add your cheese quickly.

4. Roll up and skewer your roll. Let your bacon crisp and allow your cheese to melt a little bit.

5. Serve!

Nutritional Value:

135 Calories.

9 grams of Protein.

0 grams of Carbs.

12 grams of Fat.

Mashed Rutabagas (Serves 4)

Ingredients:

2 slices of Bacon

4 ounces of Shredded Cheddar Cheese

14 ounces of Peeled & Cubed Rutabagas

4 tablespoons of Butter

8 tablespoons of Sour Cream

Directions:

1. Peel and cube your rutabaga.

2. Place it in your pan and cover it with your water.

3. Boil them and reduce down to a simmer.

4. Fry up two slices of bacon while your rutabaga cook.

5. Place your rutabagas in your food processor and mix.

6. Add your sour cream, butter, and cheese. Process some more.

7. Fold in your crumbled bacon using a spatula.

8. Serve!

Nutritional Value:

334 Calories.

11 grams of Protein.

9 grams of Carbs.

28 grams of Fat.

Cheddar Garlic Biscuits (Serves 37)

Ingredients:

6 ounces of Shredded Colby Jack Cheese

2 Large Eggs

2 teaspoons of Granulated Garlic

2 1/2 cups of Almond Flour

8 ounces of Cream Cheese

5 tablespoons of Butter

3/4 teaspoon of Xanthan Gum

1 teaspoon of Baking Soda

1 teaspoon of Sea Salt

Directions:

1. Preheat your oven to 325 degrees and line your cookie sheet with some parchment paper.

2. In your food processor place your shredded cheese and 1 cup of almond flour. Process until finely grained. Put to the side.

3. In your glass mixing bowl, place your cream cheese and butter. Microwave for 30 seconds. Whisk until glossy and smooth.

4. Whisk in your eggs until it is smooth. Mix in your baking soda, garlic, salt, and xanthan gum.

5. Add your almond flour cheese mix to egg mixture. Add your remaining almond flour and fold in until it is mixed together well and a dough begins forming.

6. Drop mixture by tablespoon onto your cookie sheet. Space each an inch apart. Roll dough a bit to smooth it out so it makes a prettier biscuit.

7. Bake approximately 20 to 25 minutes. Should be golden brown on top. Remove and allow it to cool down for 10 minutes. Makes approximately 37 biscuits.

8. Serve!

Nutritional Value:

96 Calories.

3 grams of Protein.

2 grams of Carbs.

9 grams of Fat.

Turnip Hash Browns (Serves 2)

Ingredients:

1 Rutabaga

1 Large Egg

2 ounces of Shredded Cheese

2 tablespoons of Bacon Grease

Onion Powder

Granulated Garlic

Salt

Pepper

Directions:

1. Peel and quarter your rutabaga. Shred 4 ounces of rutabaga.

2. Combine your cheese and egg with rutabaga. Mix together well.

3. Heat your bacon grease in your skillet.

4. Add your mixture. Cook for a few minutes turning it once.

5. Serve!

Nutritional Value:

231 Calories.

8 grams of Protein.

6 grams of Carbs.

20 grams of Fat.

Kale & Bacon Chips

Ingredients:

1 bunch of Kale

2 tablespoons of Butter

1/4 cup of Bacon Grease

2 teaspoons of Salt

Garlic Powder

Directions:

1. Preheat your oven to approximately 300 degrees. Line your cookie sheet with some parchment paper.

2. Remove leaves from kale. Tear kale into smaller bit sized pieces. Wash and dry thoroughly.

3. Add your butter to bacon grease and warm until in a liquid state. Add in your salt and stir.

4. Put kale in a gallon sized Ziploc bag. Add your liquid butter and bacon grease mixture. Don't completely seal the bag. You have to be able to shake kale leaves around so they can get completely coated. You want the leaves shiny green. No dry leaves.

5. Pour your bag onto your cookie sheet. Make sure leaves are all in a single layer and completely coated. Sprinkle with your garlic powder.

6. Bake approximately 20 to 25 minutes until the leaves turn dark green and get crispy but not burnt.

7. Serve!

Nutritional Value:

62 Calories.

1 gram of Protein.

1 gram of Carbs.

6 grams of Fat.

Sauteed Cauliflower

Ingredients:

9 ounces of Cauliflower

1 tablespoon of Bacon Grease

Salt

Pepper

Directions:

1. Boil your cauliflower for approximately 5 to 10 minutes.

2. Squeeze any liquid out of your cauliflower using your potato ricer.

3. Fry it in your bacon grease. Season with salt and pepper when your almost finished cooking.

4. Serve!

Sauteed Mushrooms (Serves 2)

Ingredients:

10 ounces of White Button Mushrooms

3 tablespoons of Bacon Grease

1 teaspoon of Parmesan Cheese

Garlic

Salt

Pepper

Directions:

1. Slice your mushrooms.

2. Cook your mushrooms with bacon grease in your skillet.

3. Season with your garlic powder, pepper, and salt.

4. Grate your Parmesan cheese onto your mushrooms.

5. Serve!

Nutritional Value:

185 Calories.

4 grams of Protein.

4 grams of Carbs.

17 grams of Fat.

Bacon Wrapped Smokies

Ingredients:

45 Smokies / Cocktail Wieners

10 slices of Bacon

45 Toothpicks

Directions:

1. Cut your bacon into 3 or 4 strips.

2. Wrap each of your wieners with a slice of bacon and spear it with one toothpick.

3. Cook at 400 degrees until done. Finish them off with your broiler.

Bacon Wrapped Asparagus

Ingredients:

8 slices of Bacon

40 spears of Asparagus

Directions:

1. Wash your asparagus.

2. Bend each asparagus and break at a weak point. Throw out the base part.

3. Make a bundle of 5 asparagus spears and wrap with one piece of bacon.

4. Bake it at 400 degrees until it is done. Finish them off with your broiler.

Coffee Smoothie (Serves 2)

Ingredients:

6 ounces of Cold Coffee

2 tablespoons of Unsweetened Cocoa

4 ounces of Unsweetened Milk

4 ounces of Heavy Cream

1 ounce of Torani Sugar-Free Chocolate Syrup

1 ounce of Torani Sugar-Free Caramel Syrup

16 ounces of Ice

Directions:

1. Add your liquids to your blender, then add your powder and your ice.

2. Use the smoothie setting on Vitamix with your tamper attachment to push your mix towards blades.

3. Serve!

Nutritional Value:

216 Calories.

3 grams of Protein.

6 grams of Carbs.

22 grams of Fat.

Avocado Shake (Serves 1)

Ingredients:

3 ounces of Heavy Whipping Cream

1 Avocado

6 drops of EZ-Sweetz

3 ounces of Unsweetened Almond Milk

6 Ice Cubes

Directions:

1. Add your almond milk, EZ-Sweetz, and heavy whipping cream to your Vitamix.

2. Cut your avocado in half and remove the seed. Remove the flesh from the skin and add to your mixer.

3. Add in your 6 ice cubes.

4. Blend on your smoothie setting. For regular blender keep blending until your mixture has a yogurt consistency.

5. Serve!

Nutritional Value:

587 Calories.

6 grams of Protein.

18 grams of Carbs.

58 grams of Fat.

Raspberry Lemonade Poptail (Serves 2)

Ingredients:

2 ounces of Heavy Cream

1/3 ounce of Lemon Juice

2/3 ounce of Vodka

4/5 ounce of Torani Sugar-Free Raspberry Syrup

1/4 ounce of Vanilla

Directions:

1. Freeze your Zoku device 24 hours until fully frozen.

2. Each popsicle uses 2 ounces of your total mix.

3. Mix your ingredients and then place in your freezer.

4. Bring out your Zoku device and place your popsicle stick into it.

5. Add your liquid and wait for approximately 16 minutes. May take a little longer to freeze due to the alcohol in it.

6. Once completely frozen, screw on your extractor and release from the mold.

7. Snap your drip shield on.

8. Serve!

Nutritional Value:

125 Calories.

0 grams of Protein.

1 grams of Carbs.

10 grams of Fat.

White Russian Poptail (Serves 2)

Ingredients:

2/3 ounce of Unsweetened Coconut Milk

2 ounces of Heavy Cream

2/3 ounce of Da Vinci Sugar-Free Kahlua Syrup

2/3 ounce of Vodka

Directions:

1. Freeze your Zoku device 24 hours until it is fully frozen.

2. Each popsicle uses 2 ounces of your total mix.

3. Mix your ingredients and then place in your freezer.

4. Bring out your Zoku device and place your popsicle stick into it.

5. Add your liquid and wait for approximately 16 minutes. May take a little longer to freeze due to the alcohol in it.

6. Once completely frozen, screw on your extractor and release from the mold.

7. Snap your drip shield on.

8. Serve!

Nutritional Value:

125 Calories.

0 grams of Protein.

1 gram of Carbs.

10 grams of Fat.

Alcohol-Infused Whipped Cream (Serves 10)

Ingredients:

6 3/4 ounces of Heavy Cream

1 2/3 ounces of Vanilla Vodka

1/4 teaspoon of EZ-Sweetz

1/4 teaspoon of Vanilla

Directions:

1. Combine all your ingredients and place in your iSi Mini Easy Whip Container.

2. Charge it with your nitrogen cartridge.

3. Shake 3 to 4 times, if it comes out a little runny just shake some more.

4. Pour into your bowl or on top of your drink or dessert.

5. Serve!

Nutritional Value:

23 Calories.

0 grams of Protein.

0 grams of Carbs.

1 gram of Fat.

Keto Apple Martini (Serves 1)

Ingredients:

2 ounces of Plain Vodka

1 teaspoon of Low-Carb Sugar Syrup

2 ounces of Apple Flavored Vodka

Apple slice

Directions:

1. Finely dice your apple slice and place it in your cocktail shaker.

2. Add your sugar syrup and then mash them both together.

3. Add both types of your vodka and ice. Shake it well.

4. Strain it into your martini glass.

5. Serve!

Blueberry Martini (Serves 1)

Ingredients:

2 ounces of Blueberry Flavored Vodka

2 ounces of Plain Vodka

7 Fresh Blueberries

1 teaspoon of Low-Carb Sugar Syrup

Directions:

1. Place your blueberries in your cocktail shaker.

2. Add your sugar syrup and then mash them both together.

3. Add both types of your vodka and ice. Shake it well.

4. Strain it into your martini glass.

5. Serve!

Low Carb Keto Mojito (Serves 1)

Ingredients:

2 1/2 ounces of Light Rum

8 Mint Leaves w/ Stems

1 tablespoon of Low-Carb Sugar Syrup

1 Lime

Club Soda

Directions:

1. Finely dice your mint leaves and mix with your sugar syrup using a tall glass.

2. Cut your lime in half. Discard your seeds. Squeeze juice from both halves into your glass.

3. Add your rum and stir.

4. Add your ice and club soda.

5. Serve!

Low Carb Keto Pina Colada (Serves 2)

Ingredients:

3 ounces of Rum

1/2 cup of Sugar-Free Pineapple Syrup

2/3 cup of Sugar-Free Cream or Coconut Milk

2 cups of Crushed Ice

Directions:

1. Add your ingredients to your blender and mix until they get slushy.

2. Pour equally into 2 glasses.

3. Serve!

Keto Raspberry Vinaigrette

Ingredients:

1/2 cup of Golden Raspberries

1/2 cup of White Wine Vinegar

1/2 cup of Extra Virgin Olive Oil

35 drops of Liquid Stevia

Directions:

1. Combine your olive oil, vinegar, and liquid stevia into your container that you can fit in an immersion blender.

2. Add your raspberries to a container and blend it well using your immersion blender.

3. Strain your seeds out from vinaigrette, saving the liquid portion. Pour on top of your salad.

4. Serve!

Nutritional Value:

84 Calories.

0.1 grams of Protein.

0.3 grams of Carbs.

9.3 grams of Fat.

Simple Bleu Cheese Dressing (Serves 2)

Ingredients:

2 ounces of Mayo

1 ounce of Sour Cream

3 ounces of Bleu Cheese

1 ounce of Cream Cheese

1/2 tablespoon of Lemon Juice

Directions:

1. Add your 2 ounces of bleu cheese and the rest of your ingredients into your immersion blender.

2. Run your blender until finely grated.

3. Once you've blended it, crumble in your remaining 1 ounce of bleu cheese.

4. Serve!

Nutritional Value:

401 Calories.

12 grams of Protein.

2 grams of Carbs.

38 grams of Fat.

Keto Blackberry Chipotle Jam (Serves 10)

Ingredients:

8 ounces of Blackberries

1/4 cup of MCT Oil

8 drops of Liquid Stevia

1 1/2 Chipotle in Adobo

1/4 teaspoon of Guar Gum

1/4 cup of Erythritol

Directions:

1. Add your blackberries to your pan over a low heat. Allow it to cook slightly so it becomes soft. Cook for approximately 5 minutes.

2. Add your chipotle in adobo to your mixture.

3. Add your erythritol and the stevia to your pan and mix into blackberries. Crush your blackberries using a fork and mix together.

4. Add your MCT Oil to your pan and turn the heat to medium. Allow your jam to boil, reduce the heat to low and allow it to simmer for 6 to 8 minutes.

5. Add your guar gum to jam and mix well. Continue to mix it for approximately 1 to 2 minutes until the mixture thickens.

6. Strain your seeds from jam using colander and back of metal spoon. Discard the seeds when done.

7. Serve!

Nutritional Value:

51 Calories.

0.3 grams of Protein.

1.1 grams of Carbs.

5.7 grams of Fat.

Horseradish Sauce (Serves 8)

Ingredients:

1/4 cup of Sour Cream

3/4 tablespoon of Prepared Horseradish

1 teaspoon of Dijon Mustard

1 tablespoon of Mayo

Directions:

1. Mix your ingredients together and then serve cold.

Nutritional Value:

30 Calories.

0 grams of Protein.

1 grams of Carbs.

3 grams of Fat.

Keto Caesar Dressing (Serves 8)

Ingredients:

3 cloves of Minced Garlic

1 1/2 teaspoons of Dijon Mustard

1 1/2 teaspoons of Anchovy Paste

3/4 cup of Mayo

2 tablespoons of Fresh Lemon Juice

1 teaspoon of Worcestershire Sauce

Salt

Pepper

Directions:

1. Mince your garlic cloves and use your garlic press. Add to your large-sized bowl.

2. Add your anchovy paste, lemon juice, Worcestershire sauce, and Dijon mustard to your garlic and whisk it all together.

3. Add your mayonnaise to your bowl and whisk until it's all combined.

4. Serve!

Nutritional Value:

140 Calories.

0.1 grams of Protein.

0.8 grams of Carbs.

15.1 grams of Fat.

Chapter Five: Ketogenic Diet Dessert Recipes

In this section, I will give you 30+ keto dessert recipes you can make yourself. I'll include both basic recipes and a few more advanced recipes. That way no matter what your level is in the kitchen you'll be able to prepare yourself a healthy low-carb ketogenic dessert to keep you on track with your diet. I'll add in the nutritional value whenever possible, although I don't always have those exact numbers for each and every recipe.

Chocolate Chia Pudding (Serves 2)

Ingredients:

3 tablespoons of Chia Seeds

1/4 cup of Fresh or Frozen Raspberries

1 scoop of Chocolate Protein Powder or Cocoa Powder

1 cup of Unsweetened Almond Milk or Skim Milk

1 teaspoon of Honey (Only If Not Using The Protein Powder)

Directions:

1. Mix your chocolate protein powder and almond milk together. Make sure you've stirred it well.

2. Add in your chia seeds. Make sure you've stirred it in well.

3. Allow your mix to rest for approximately 5 minutes and then stir.

4. Stir again approximately 5 minutes later.

5. Allow your mix to rest for approximately 30 minutes in your refrigerator.

6. Add your raspberries on the top.

7. Serve!

Nutritional Value:

235 Calories.

30 grams of Protein.

19 grams of Carbs.

12 grams of Fat.

Coconut Butter Cup Fat Bombs (Serves 4)

Ingredients:

4 tablespoons of Cocoa Powder

4 teaspoons of Coconut Butter

4 tablespoons of Coconut Oil

2 tablespoons of Erythritol

Pinch of Salt

Directions:

1. Combine your cocoa powder, erythritol, and coconut oil. Stir until no clumps are left. Add a pinch of salt.

2. Warm up your coconut butter if not soft enough.

3. Pour half of your chocolate mixture into 4 silicone cupcake molds evenly. Tilt each mold so the chocolate will coat the edge a bit. Place in your freezer for approximately 5 minutes.

4. When this has hardened, spoon a teaspoon of your coconut butter into each of your molds. Spread them evenly on each mold so it covers the entire chocolate layer. Place in your freezer for approximately 5 minutes.

5. Take your remaining half of chocolate mix and use it to cover the hardened coconut butter layer. Spread evenly. Freeze again for approximately 5 minutes.

6. Serve!

Nutritional Value:

260 Calories.

3 grams of Protein.

0.5 grams of Carbs.

26 grams of Fat.

Jalapeno Popper Fat Bombs (Serves 3)

Ingredients:

3 ounces of Cream Cheese

1 Medium Jalapeno Pepper

3 slices of Bacon

1/2 teaspoon of Dried Parsley

1/4 teaspoon of Garlic Powder

1/4 teaspoon of Onion Powder

Pepper

Salt

Directions:

1. Fry 3 slices of your bacon in a pan until it is crisp.

2. Remove your bacon from the pan, but keep the remaining grease for later use. Wait until your bacon is cooked and crisp.

3. De-seed your jalapeno pepper, then dice into small pieces.

4. Combine your cream cheese, jalapeno, and spices. Season with your salt and pepper.

5. Add your bacon fat in and mix together until a solid mixture is formed.

6. Crumble your bacon and set on a plate. Roll your cream cheese mixture into balls using your hand, then roll the ball into your bacon.

7. Serve!

Nutritional Value:

207 Calories.

5 grams of Protein.

1.5 grams of Carbs.

19 grams of Fat.

Neapolitan Fat Bombs (Serves 24)

Ingredients:

1/2 cup of Butter

2 Medium Strawberries

1/2 cup of Coconut Oil

1/2 cup of Cream Cheese

1/2 cup of Sour Cream

2 tablespoons of Cocoa Powder

2 tablespoons of Erythritol

1 teaspoon of Vanilla Extract

25 drops of Liquid Stevia

Directions:

1. In your bowl, combine your butter, coconut oil, sour cream, cream cheese, erythritol, and liquid stevia.

2. Using an immersion blender, blend together your ingredients into a smooth mixture.

3. Divide your mixture into 3 different bowls. Add cocoa powder to one bowl, strawberries to another bowl, and vanilla to the last bowl.

4. Mix together all of your ingredients again using an immersion blender. Separate your chocolate mixture into a container with a spout.

5. Pour your chocolate mixture into a fat bomb mold. Place in your freezer for 30 minutes, then repeat with your vanilla mixture.

6. Freeze your vanilla mixture for 30 minutes, then repeat the process with strawberry mixture. Freeze again for at least 1 hour.

7. Once they're completely frozen, remove from your fat bomb molds.

8. Serve!

Nutritional Value:

102 Calories.

0.6 grams of Protein.

0.4 grams of Carbs.

11 grams of Fat.

Chocolate Strawberry Mousse (Serves 1)

Ingredients:

1 Strawberry

1/2 scoop of Chocolate Whey Powder

1/3 cup of Heavy Whipping Cream

2 1/2 grams of Unsweetened Cocoa

4 drops of EZ-Sweet

Flakes of 90% Chocolate

Directions:

1. Measure your cream into your container.

2. Add your EZ-Sweet.

3. Add your strawberry.

4. Add your powder.

5. Add your chocolate flakes.

6. Mix 1 to 2 minutes until stiff.

7. Serve!

Nutritional Value:

330 Calories.

10 grams of Protein.

12 grams of Carbs.

33 grams of Fat.

Peanut Butter Cookies (Serves 15)

Ingredients:

1 Egg

1 cup of Peanut Butter

1/2 cup of Powdered Erythritol

Directions:

1. Preheat your oven to 350 degrees.

2. Combine your ingredients and mix together well.

3. Roll your mix into 1-inch balls and place on your baking sheet lined with parchment paper.

4. Bake for approximately 10 to 15 minutes until the cookie edges begin to turn dark brown.

5. Allow to cool on wire rack.

6. Serve!

Nutritional Value:

105 Calories.

4 grams of Protein.

2 grams of Carbs.

9 grams of Fat.

Cake Batter Cookies (Serves 12)

Ingredients:

Cookies:

1/4 cup of Softened Butter

1/4 cup of Erythritol

1 Egg

1 Egg Yolk

1 cup of Sukrin Gold

1 1/2 teaspoons of Butter Extract

3/4 cup of Almond Flour

1 teaspoon of Vanilla Extract

1/4 teaspoon of Almond Extract

1 tablespoon of Coconut Flour

1/2 teaspoon of Xanthan Gum

2 tablespoons of Rainbow Sprinkles

1/2 teaspoon of Salt

Optional Filling:

1/4 cup of Softened Butter

1/2 cup of Sukrin Melis

Directions:

1. Cream together your erythritol, Sukrin Gold, and softened butter with your electric hand mixer.

2. Mix in your egg yolk and egg.

3. Add your butter, almond, and vanilla extracts.

4. Add your salt and flours. Mix it well until it is combined.

5. Add your xanthan gum. Mix until your batter thickens.

6. Mix in your sprinkles and stir to evenly distribute them.

7. Refrigerate your batter for a little bit.

8. Lay out saran wrap and place your cookie batter onto it.

9. Wrap your batter into log 3-inches thick. Make sure the thickness is uniform throughout. Refrigerate 2 hours to allow to harden.

10. Take out of your refrigerator and preheat your oven to 350 degrees. Unwrap your log and roll to get rid of flattened edges. Slice your log into desired cookie thickness. For this example, I cut them into 12 cookies.

11. Line your cookies on a baking sheet lined with parchment paper and cook for approximately 10 minutes. Cookies are done when slightly golden.

12. Allow your cookies to cool down.

13. You can make the optional filling above combining two ingredients. Then put on top of a cookie and place another cookie on top making into a cookie sandwich.

14. Serve!

Nutritional Value:

175 Calories.

3 grams of Protein.

2 grams of Carbs.

17 grams of Fat.

Keto Mug Cookie (Serves 1)

Ingredients:

1 Egg Yolk

1 tablespoon of Erythritol

1 tablespoon of Butter

1/8 teaspoon of Vanilla Extract

3 tablespoons of Almond Flour

2 tablespoons of Sugar-Free Chocolate Chips

Pinch of Salt

Pinch of Cinnamon

Directions:

1. Preheat your oven to 350 degrees.

2. Melt your butter in a small-sized pan and allow it to brown a bit.

3. Combine your butter with almond flour.

4. Add in your cinnamon and erythritol.

5. Add your vanilla extract, egg yolk, and salt.

6. Spray cup or mug with cooking oil and place in your mixture. Flatten it out to make sure it cooks evenly.

7. Press into your cup.

8. Microwave for 1 minute on high or bake in your oven approximately 10 minutes.

9. Allow it to cool.

10. Serve!

Nutritional Value:

330 Calories.

7 grams of Protein.

3 grams of Carbs.

31 grams of Fat.

Coconut Macaroons (Serves 10)

Ingredients:

4 Egg Whites

1/2 teaspoon of EZ-Sweet

1 teaspoon of Vanilla

2 cups of Unsweetened Coconut

4 1/2 teaspoons of Water

Directions:

1. Combine your egg whites and liquids.

2. Add in your coconut and mix together.

3. Spread on your greased pie pan.

4. Preheat your oven to 375 degrees. When you put in your macaroons reduce the heat to 325 degrees and bake for approximately 14 minutes.

5. Serve!

Nutritional Value:

88 Calories.

2 grams of Protein.

3 grams of Carbs.

8 grams of Fat.

Butter Pecan Ice Cream (Serves 6)

Ingredients:

2 Egg Yolks

1/3 cup of Erythritol

1 cup of Heavy Cream

1 teaspoon of Vanilla Extract

2 tablespoons of Butter

1/8 teaspoon of Xanthan Gum

2/3 cups of Chopped Pecans

Pinch of Stevia

Directions:

1. Melt your butter in your pan over a low flame. Allow it to brown slightly.

2. Add in your cream and allow it to simmer.

3. Turn your heat to the lowest setting, adding your erythritol. Allow it to completely dissolve. Stir gently.

4. Transfer your mixture into your large-sized mixing bowl. Add your Stevia. Use your electric hand mixer to get your ingredients combined.

5. While mixing on the medium setting, add your xanthan gum to allow your ingredients to thicken and bind.

6. In another small-sized bowl, separate your egg yolks and add in your vanilla extract. Slowly beat them into your mixing bowl as you're beating the cream mixture.

7. Add your chopped pecans and fold in using a spoon.

8. Place your bowl in your freezer. Take out to stir every 40 minutes so pecans are well incorporated.

9. Allow it to freeze for at least 3 hours before serving.

10. Serve!

Nutritional Value:

200 Calories.

2 grams of Protein.

1 gram of Carbs.

20 grams of Fat.

Strawberry Swirl Ice Cream (Serves 6)

Ingredients:

3 Large Egg Yolks

1/3 cup of Erythritol

1 cup of Heavy Cream

1 cup of Pureed Strawberries

1/2 teaspoon of Vanilla Extract

1 tablespoon of Vodka (Optional)

1/8 teaspoon of Xanthan Gum (Optional)

Directions:

1. Set a pot with your heavy cream over a low flame to heat up. Add in your erythritol.

2. Don't let your cream boil, just let it gently simmer until your erythritol is all dissolved.

3. Separate your egg yolks into your large-sized mixing bowl. Beat with your electric mixer until doubled in size.

4. Temper your eggs so they don't scramble, add a couple of tablespoons of the heated cream mixture at a time to the eggs while you're beating them.

5. Continue until your egg mixture is warm and then add in the rest of your cream mixture slowly, beating them constantly.

6. Add in your vanilla extract and mix.

7. Optional step. Add in your vodka and xanthan gum.

8. Place your bowl in your freezer and leave for 2 hours occasionally taking out to stir, Can also churn using your ice cream maker if you have one.

9. Puree your strawberries.

10. Once the ice cream has been chilled and is beginning to thicken add in your pureed strawberries.

11. Mix in your strawberries but don't mix too much. You want ribbons of your strawberry visible in the ice cream.

12. Place in your freezer for 4 to 6 hours.

13. Serve!

Nutritional Value:

178 Calories.

2.3 grams of Protein.

2.8 grams of Carbs.

16.9 grams of Fat.

Mint Chocolate Chip Ice Cream (Serves 4)

Ingredients:

1 cup of Heavy Cream

1/2 teaspoon of Liquid Stevia Extract

1/2 cup of Light Cream

1 Square Dark Chocolate (Optional)

1/2 teaspoon of Vanilla (Optional)

Several drops of Peppermint Extract (Optional)

Several drops of Green Food Coloring (Optional)

Directions:

1. Place your ice cream bowl in your freezer 4 to 12 hours ahead of time.

2. Place all of your ingredients in your ice cream bowl except the chocolate.

3. Whisk together well.

4. Place in your freezer for approximately 5 minutes.

5. Set up your ice cream maker and add in liquid.

6. Make ice cream according to your machine's instructions. A few minutes before ice cream sets, add in your chocolate shavings.

7. Store in your air tight container and place back in your freezer.

8. Allow it to freeze.

9. Serve!

Nutritional Value:

295 Calories.

2.25 grams of Protein.

3.5 grams of Carbs.

31 grams of Fat.

Chocolate Chip Peanut Butter Ice Cream

Ingredients:

3 Large Egg Yolks

3/4 cup of Sugar-Free Chocolate Chips

1/2 cup of Heavy Cream

1/2 cup of Almond Milk

1/2 cup of Peanut Butter

1/4 cup of Erythritol

1 teaspoon of Vanilla Extract

1/4 teaspoon of Xanthan Gum

1 tablespoon of Vodka (Optional)

Directions:

1. Heat your erythritol and heavy cream on a stove over a low heat. Don't boil. Allow it to come to a gentle simmer.

2. While that's heating up, whisk together your egg yolks and add in your vanilla extract.

3. Temper your eggs so they don't scramble by slowly adding hot cream while continuing to whisk.

4. Pour your tempered eggs into your hot cream and whisk over a low flame.

5. Add in your xanthan gum and mix until everything thickens up.

6. Transfer to your bowl and add your vodka if you're using it. Chill until it is cooled down.

7. Once your mixture is cool, add to your ice cream maker and follow the instructions for that machine.

8. Once your ice cream is thick in your ice cream maker, add your chocolate chips. In last few seconds of churning, add in your peanut butter.

9. Place in your freezer if you want it harder.

10. Serve!

Nutritional Value:

295 Calories.

8 grams of Protein.

5.8 grams of Carbs.

26 grams of Fat.

Keto Strawberry Cheesecake (Serves 8)

Ingredients:

Crust:

4 tablespoons of Butter

3/4 cup of Pecans

3/4 cup of Almond Flour

2 tablespoons of Splenda

Filling:

4 Eggs

1 1/2 pounds of Cream Cheese

9 Strawberries

1/2 tablespoon of Liquid Vanilla

1/2 tablespoon of Lemon Juice

1/2 teaspoon of EZ-Sweetz

1/4 cup of Sour Cream

Directions:

1. Preheat your oven to approximately 400 degrees.

2. Crush up your pecans.

3. In your small-sized saucepan, melt your butter and add in your almond flour, pecans, and Splenda.

4. Mix your crust in your saucepan for several minutes until your ingredients are combined.

5. Grease your 9-inch springform pan. Line the bottom with your crust mixture.

6. Cook at 400 degrees approximately 7 minutes until your crust begins to brown.

7. Combine all of your filling ingredients in a stand mixer and combine well.

8. Slice some additional strawberries and line side of crust if you'd like.

9. Add your filling on top of your crust.

10. Top with more strawberries if you'd like.

11. Put your cheesecake in your oven and drop it from 400 degrees to 250 degrees as soon as it's in the oven.

12. Cook for approximately 60 to 90 minutes until your cheesecake has set.

13. Allow it to cool.

14. Serve!

Nutritional Value:

535 Calories.

13 grams of Protein.

9 grams of Carbs.

49 grams of Fat.

Red Velvet Cinnamon Cheesecakes (Serves 4)

Ingredients:

Red Velvet Layer:

1 Egg

1 tablespoon of Cocoa Powder

1/4 cup of Butter

1/2 teaspoon of Apple Cider Vinegar

1 teaspoon of Red Food Coloring

6 tablespoons of Almond Flour

1/2 teaspoon of Vanilla Extract

Pinch of Salt

Cheesecake Layer:

1 Egg

1 tablespoon of Butter

6 ounces of Cream Cheese

1/2 teaspoon of Vanilla Extract

2 tablespoons of Erythritol

1 teaspoon of Cinnamon

Pinch of Salt

Directions:

Red Velvet Layer:

1. Preheat your oven to 350 degrees.

2. Melt your butter in your small-sized saucepan. Combine it with your erythritol. Keep the flame on a low heat until your erythritol is dissolved.

3. In your mixing bowl, combine your butter and erythritol with salt, vanilla, and cocoa powder.

4. Add in your egg and mix together until it is well combined.

5. Add in your food coloring and your apple cider vinegar.

6. Add your sifted almond flour and mix it together until fully combined.

7. Evenly pour your mixture among 4 greased ramekins. Be sure to tap a hard surface to flatten your batter out and remove the air bubbles. Place them on your cookie sheet and place them into your refrigerator while you're making your cheesecake layer.

Cheesecake Layer:

8. Using your electric hand mixer, beat your softened cream cheese and butter until light and fluffy.

9. Add in your vanilla extract, cinnamon, and egg. Beat your mixture again.

10. Add your powdered erythritol and salt. Mix with your electric hand mixer.

Combining:

11. Take your ramekins out of your refrigerator and spoon about 2 big teaspoons onto each of your red velvet layers. They shouldn't mix but should meet without having any gaps between each of them.

12. Use your spoon to push the cheesecake layer to edges of your ramekins. Make sure there are no gaps between your ramekins and your cakes. Tap your ramekins again on a hard surface so your top layer will flatten out.

13. Bake in your oven for approximately 20 minutes. Make sure tops are set before removing from oven.

14. Allow it to cool.

15. Serve!

Nutritional Value:

420 Calories.

17 grams of Protein.

2 grams of Carbs.

36 grams of Fat.

No Bake Lemon Cheesecake

Ingredients:

8 ounces of Softened Cream Cheese

2 ounces of Heavy Cream

1 teaspoon of Stevia Glycerite

1 tablespoon of Lemon Juice

1 teaspoon of Vanilla Flavoring

1 teaspoon of Splenda

Directions:

1. Mix all your ingredients together and then whip it into a pudding-like consistency. Spoon your mixture into small-sized serving cups and then refrigerate until it sets.

2. Serve!

White Chocolate Raspberry Cheesecake Fluff

Ingredients:

8 ounces of Softened Cream Cheese

1 teaspoon of Low Sugar Raspberry Preserves

2 ounces of Heavy Cream

1 tablespoon of Da Vinci Sugar-Free White Chocolate Flavor Syrup

1 teaspoon of Stevia Glycerite

Directions:

1. Mix all your ingredients together and then whip it into a pudding-like consistency. Spoon your mixture into small-sized serving cups and then refrigerate until it sets.

2. Serve!

Chocolate Chip Cheesecake

Ingredients:

8 ounces of Softened Cream Cheese

2 ounces of Heavy Cream

1 teaspoon of Splenda

1 ounce of Mini Chocolate Chips

1 teaspoon of Stevia Glycerite

Directions:

1. Mix all your ingredients together and then whip it into a pudding-like consistency. Spoon your mixture into small-sized serving cups and then refrigerate until it sets.

2. Serve!

Double Chocolate Bundt Cake (Serves 8)

Ingredients:

Bundt Cake:

3 Large Eggs

2 cups of Anthony's Almond Flour

1 cup of Butter

1 1/2 teaspoons of Baking Soda

2 tablespoons of Coconut Flour

1 cup of Erythritol

1 cup of Water

1/2 cup of Sour Cream

1/2 cup of Cocoa Powder

2 teaspoons of Vanilla Extract

1/2 teaspoon of Salt

White Chocolate Glaze:

2 tablespoons of Heavy Cream

1 teaspoon of Vanilla Extract

2 ounces of Anthony's Organic Cocoa Butter Wafers

3 tablespoons of Powdered Erythritol

Topping:

20 grams of Anthony's Organic Cocoa Nibs

Directions:

1. Preheat your oven to 350 degrees.

2. Whisk together 2 cups of Anthony's Blanched Almond Flour with your baking soda, salt, coconut flour, and erythritol.

3. Heat up your butter, water, and cocoa powder in your small-sized pot over a medium heat. Whisk until it is combined and then take off heat.

4. Pour half the chocolate mixture into your dry mix and stir it to combine. Once it thickens, pour in other half and stir to combine again.

5. Add 1 egg at a time to your mixture.

6. Add your vanilla extract and sour cream. Stir well.

7. Pour your mixture into a greased bundt cake pan. Bake for approximately 40 to 50 minutes.

8. Prepare glaze while cake bakes. Melt your cocoa butter wafers.

9. Add your powdered erythritol and stir to combine. Add your heavy cream and place in refrigerator. Take out and stir approximately every 5 minutes.

10. Once opaque and thick, pulse it using your Nutribullet or blend in your blender until it is smooth.

11. Once cake is done baking, allow it to cool in its pan for approximately 10 minutes. Invert onto a cooling rack on your baking sheet or plate. Allow it to completely cool.

12. Glaze your cake. While glaze is wet, sprinkle your cocoa nibs over your cake. Allow the glaze to cool down and harden.

13. Serve!

Nutritional Value:

520 Calories.

10 grams of Protein.

5 grams of Carbs.

50 grams of Fat.

Chocolate Caramel Lave Cake (Serves 4)

Ingredients:

1/2 cup of Cocoa Powder

1/8 teaspoon of Powdered Stevia

1/4 cup of Carolyn's Low-Carb Caramel Sauce

4 Medium Eggs

1/4 cup of Erythritol

1/4 cup of Melted Butter

1/2 teaspoon of Cinnamon

1 teaspoon of Vanilla Extract

1/4 teaspoon of Salt

Directions:

1. Prepare your caramel sauce and allow it to cool. Put some in a small-sized jar and allow it to freeze.

2. Preheat your oven to 350 degrees.

3. Prepare your lava cake batter. Combine all your dry ingredients and mix to get out lumps.

4. Combine your wet ingredients and mix with your dry ingredients.

5. Spray your 4 ramekins with oil or use some butter to grease them.

6. Fill your ramekins halfway each with your batter.

7. Place a tablespoon of caramel sauce into center of each of your ramekin, letting it rest on your lava cake batter.

8. Pour rest of your batter over caramel. Cover it completely.

9. Place your ramekins on your baking sheet and bake for approximately 13 minutes. Tops of cake should be set but still jiggle.

10. Allow it to relax for approximately 3 minutes. Run a sharp knife around edges of the ramekin to loosen your cakes.

11. Place your plate upside down onto your ramekin. Flip your ramekin and plate so your ramekin is now facing upside down on your plate. Tap your ramekin to make your cake gently fall onto your plate.

12. Add your desired optional toppings.

13. Serve!

Nutritional Value:

230 Calories.

8 grams of Protein.

6 grams of Carbs.

24 grams of Fat.

Keto Lava Cake (Serves 1)

Ingredients:

1 Medium Egg

2 tablespoons of Cocoa Powder

2 tablespoons of Erythritol

1 tablespoon of Heavy Cream

1/4 teaspoon of Baking Powder

1/2 teaspoon of Vanilla Extract

Pinch of Salt

Directions:

1. Preheat your oven to 350 degrees.

2. Combine your cocoa powder and erythritol. Mix until it is smooth. Remove any clumps that form.

3. In a separate bowl, beat your egg until fluffy.

4. Add your heavy cream, vanilla extract, and egg to your cocoa mixture. Add your baking soda and salt.

5. Spray your cooking oil into your mug and pour your batter in. Bake for approximately 10 to 15 minutes at 350 degrees. The top should be set but still jiggly.

6. Allow to relax for approximately 3 minutes. Run your sharp knife around edges of the ramekin to loosen your cakes.

7. Place your plate upside down onto your mug. Flip your mug and plate so mug is now facing upside down on your plate. Tap mug to make your cake gently fall onto your plate.

8. Add your desired optional toppings. I like to add a scoop of ice cream on top.

9. Serve!

Nutritional Value:

173 Calories.

8 grams of Protein.

4 grams of Carbs.

13 grams of Fat.

Pink Lemonade Cloud Cake (Serves 2)

Ingredients:

Layers:

1 Oopsie Roll

1/4 teaspoon of Powdered Stevia

Frosting:

2 tablespoons of Erythritol

2 Strawberries

1 teaspoon of Fresh Lemon Juice

1/3 cup of Softened Butter

1 teaspoon of Lemon Zest

1/2 teaspoon of Poppy Seeds

1 tablespoon of Heavy Cream

Pinch of Salt

Directions:

1. Make your oopsie rolls. If you want them to be sweeter add some Stevia to your batter while making them.

2. Once cooked and you've allowed it to cool, use a mug to stamp out uniformly sized circles of your oopsie rolls.

3. Once the layers are ready, beat your erythritol and butter until it is creamy. Add a tablespoon of your cream, lemon zest, and lemon juice.

4. Add your poppy seeds and finely chopped strawberries.

5. Place your frosting mixture into a Ziploc bag and remove as much air as possible before twisting the bag and snipping the top.

6. Lay an oopsie roll on your plate and frost the outside of the cake. Follow up by filling in the middle.

7. Stack another oopsie roll on top of your frosted oopsie roll and gently press down. Repeat the previous step. Do this until you have 3 layers of oopsie rolls.

8. Garnish with your frosting and your walnut.

9. Chill in your refrigerator for approximately 1 hour.

10. Serve!

Nutritional Value:

430 Calories.

6.5 grams of Protein.

3 grams of Carbs.

42 grams of Fat.

Chocolate Covered Strawberries

Ingredients:

1/2 pound of Fresh Strawberries

1 tablespoon of Coconut Oil

2 tablespoons of Coconut Butter

2 ounces of Chocolate Chips

Directions:

1. Melt your chocolate chips. Stir well.

2. Remove from any heat and add in your coconut oil and coconut butter until everything is melted. Move to your small-sized bowl.

3. Dry your strawberries. Grab by the stem and dip into your chocolate.

4. Place your chocolate strawberries on a baking sheet lined with parchment paper and refrigerate for approximately 1 hour.

5. Serve!

Raspberry Cream Crepes

Ingredients:

Crepes:

2 Eggs

2 tablespoons of Erythritol

2 ounces of Cream Cheese

Pinch of Salt

Dash of Cinnamon

Filling:

1/2 cup + 2 tablespoons of Whole Milk Ricotta

3 ounces of Raspberries

Toppings:

Whipped Cream

Sugar-Free Maple Syrup

Directions:

1. Combine all your crepe ingredients into your food processor or blender. Blend together for approximately 20 seconds so no chunks remain.

2. Heat your pan over a medium heat. Spray with your cooking spray and put in 1/4 of your batter at a time. While pouring, tilt your pan onto all sides so your crepe batter reaches each edge of your pan.

3. Allow your crepe to cook for approximately 1 minute. Then wedge your spatula underneath and wiggle gently until you reach the center and flip it. Allow it to cook for another 15 seconds.

4. Continue doing this process until all your batter is gone. Should make 5 or 6 crepes in total.

5. Allow your crepes to cool. Lay next to one another not on top of each other.

6. Stuff them with your whole ricotta cheese.

7. Add your raspberries.

8. Fold each side of crepe over your filling and press down gently to seal it.

9. Add your toppings.

10. Serve!

Nutritional Value:

570 Calories.

15 grams of Protein.

8 grams of Carbs.

40 grams of Fat.

Pumpkin Pecan Tart (Serves 2)

Ingredients:

Crust:

1 teaspoon of Cinnamon

2 tablespoons of Melted Butter

1/2 cup of Almond Flour

Pinch of Salt

Filling:

1 Egg White

1/2 cup of Pumpkin Puree

1/4 teaspoon of Pumpkin Pie Spice

1/2 cup of Ricotta Cheese

1/2 teaspoon of Vanilla Extract

1 teaspoon of Cinnamon

2 tablespoons of Erythritol

1 Egg

Pinch of Salt

16 Pecans

Sugar-Free Maple Syrup

Directions:

1. Preheat your oven to 350 degrees. Combine your crust ingredients in your bowl.

2. Mix well and press into your mini tartlet pans. I used 4 1/2-inch pans. Allow your tart crusts to bake in your oven for approximately 10 minutes. Allow it to cool while you work on the filling.

3. Combine your egg, egg white, pumpkin puree, and ricotta cheese.

4. Mix in the rest of your filling ingredients. Stir well to combine.

5. Once your crusts are cooled, pour your filling into your crusts. Place your tart pans on a baking sheet and bake for approximately 20 minutes.

6. Remove from your oven and add pecans to top. Place back in your oven for approximately 10 minutes. The tops should have set yet still be jiggly.

7. Allow it to cool. Drizzle your maple syrup on top.

8. Serve!

Nutritional Value:

530 Calories.

19 grams of Protein.

9 grams of Carbs.

45 grams of Fat.

Pumpkin Spice Creme Brulee (Serves 2)

Ingredients:

2 Egg Yolks

2 tablespoons of Erythritol

1 cup of Heavy Cream

2 tablespoons of Pumpkin Puree

1 teaspoon of Pumpkin Pie Spice

Directions:

1. Preheat your oven to 300 degrees. Heat your heavy cream in your saucepan. Don't allow it to boil. Add in your pumpkin pie spice once your cream begins to bubble. Turn off the heat and cover with your lid. Allow it to stand for approximately 5 minutes.

2. Separate 2 egg yolks and then whisk until they're both light yellow.

3. Add some of your cream mixture a little at a time to your eggs while continuously whisking.

4. Once combined, add your pumpkin puree. Whisk together well.

5. Add in your erythritol. Mix well.

6. Place 2 ramekins in your deep baking dish and fill with hot water (approximately 1/2 way up your ramekins).

7. Pour your mixture into ramekins and bake for approximately 30 to 40 minutes. Tops of creme brulees will be set but jiggly.

8. Allow it to cool for approximately 15 minutes. Place in your refrigerator at least 4 hours.

9. Sprinkle some erythritol on top if you desire extra sweetness.

10. Use your blowtorch to burn tops of your creme brulees. Can also place in your broiler for 1 to 2 minutes if you don't have a torch.

11. Serve!

Nutritional Value:

460 Calories.

5 grams of Protein.

5 grams of Carbs.

49 grams of Fat.

Salted Caramel Panna Cotta (Serves 4)

Ingredients:

2 cups of Heavy Cream

1/4 cup of Erythritol

1 teaspoon of Vanilla

1/2 cup of Caramel

1 sachet of Unflavored Gelatin

Directions:

1. Heat up your cream in your saucepan over a low heat. Add in your erythritol and gelatin. Don't allow it to boil or simmer.

2. Use your whisk to stir together well. Add in your vanilla extract and stir well.

3. Grease your ramekins and wipe any excess with your paper towel.

4. Pour your mixture into ramekins and chill for at least 2 hours.

5. Pour 2 tablespoons of caramel over each ramekin of panna cotta.

6. Serve!

Nutritional Value:

450 Calories.

2 grams of Protein.

6 grams of Carbs.

44 grams of Fat.

Strawberry Pistachio Creamsicle (Serves 4)

Ingredients:

8 ounces of Strawberries

1/2 cup of Almond Milk

2 ounces of Salted Pistachios

1/2 cup of Heavy Cream

2 doonk scoops of Stevia

Directions:

1. Place your popsicle molds in the freezer beforehand to accelerate the freezing process.

2. Blend your heavy cream, strawberries, almond milk, and Stevia until it is fully combined. Blend for a minute.

3. Throw in your pistachios and stir. Do not blend.

4. Pour your creamsicle mix into your cold popsicle molds and insert your bases. Freeze for approximately 2 hours until it has set.

5. Remove your creamsicles by running hot water on the outside of your molds. Gently pull out.

6. Serve!

Nutritional Value:

158 Calories.

4 grams of Protein.

5.g grams of Carb.

12.5 grams of Fat.

Keto Caramel (Serves 4)

Ingredients:

4 tablespoons of Unsalted Butter

4 tablespoons of Heavy Cream

1 teaspoon of Erythritol

Pinch of Salt

Directions:

1. Melt your butter in your pan and cook until it is golden brown.

2. Pour in your heavy cream and combine. Lower your heat and simmer for approximately 1 minute.

3. Add in your erythritol. Allow it to dissolve and add your salt.

4. Cook until it gets stickier and thicker.

5. Pour into your glass container and continue to stir your caramel mixture while it cools down and thickens.

6. Serve!

Nutritional Value:

163 Calories.

0 grams of Protein.

0.5 grams of Carbs.

17 grams of Fat.

Keto Skillet Brownies (Serves 4)

Ingredients:

Brownies:

1 Egg

1/3 cup of Cocoa Powder

6 tablespoons of Butter

1/2 teaspoon of Baking Powder

1/3 cup of Erythritol

1/4 cup of Almond Flour

1/2 teaspoon of Vanilla Extract

1/4 cup of Walnuts

Pinch of Salt

Peanut Butter Drizzle:

1 tablespoon of Peanut butter

1 tablespoon of Butter

Directions:

1. Preheat your oven to 350 degrees.

2. Melt your butter in a small-sized pan and add in your erythritol. Allow it to dissolve.

3. Pour your mixture into your mixing bowl and add in your salt, vanilla extract, and cocoa powder.

4. Add in your egg and beat until it is well combined.

5. Add your baking powder and almond flour.

6. Fold in your choice of nuts. I used walnuts.

7. Pour your brownie batter into your 6-inch cast iron skillet.

8. Place in your oven and bake for approximately 30 minutes. The top will be set but still jiggly.

9. Add your peanut butter drizzle if you desire.

10. Serve!

Nutritional Value:

333 Calories.

5.8 grams of Protein.

3 grams of Carbs.

31.3 grams of Fat.

Gluten Free Banana Bread (Serves 8)

Ingredients:

Wet Ingredients:

3 Ripe Bananas

1 Juiced Orange

1/4 teaspoon of Vanilla Extract

2 tablespoons of Coconut Oil

1/4 cup of Honey

Pinch of Orange Zest

Dry Ingredients:

3/4 teaspoon of Cinnamon

1 teaspoon of Xanthan Gum

1 1/3 cup of Almond Flour

1 teaspoon of Baking Powder

1/8 teaspoon of Cayenne

1/2 teaspoon of Baking Soda

1/2 teaspoon of Salt

Fold-Ins:

2 Grated Carrots

3/4 cups of Flaxseeds

3/4 cup of Chopped Walnuts

1/4 teaspoon of Grated Fresh Ginger

Topping:

Honey

Coconut Butter

Directions:

1. Preheat your oven to 410 degrees.

2. Mash your bananas until they form a thick wet mush.

3. Add your orange zest and juiced orange.

4. Add in your vanilla extract, honey, and coconut oil.

5. Add in all your dry ingredients.

6. Shred your ginger and carrots. Fold into your mixture. Roughly chop your walnuts. Throw into your mixture.

7. Fold in the rest of your ingredients.

8. Grease your medium-sized bread pan with some butter or coconut oil. Pour in your batter. Feel free to sprinkle on sugar or drizzle some honey at the end.

9. Bake for approximately 25 minutes at 410 degrees. Lower the temperature to 350 degrees and bake for approximately 30 minutes.

10. Allow it to cool and then slice your bread.

11. Serve!

Nutritional Value:

357 Calories.

8 grams of Protein.

23 grams of Carbs.

24 grams of Fat.

Homemade Chocolate Chips (Serves 3)

Ingredients:

1 Low-Carb Chocolate Bar

Directions:

1. Melt your chocolate bar.

2 Pour your chocolate onto your silicone molds.

3. Place in your freezer and allow it to freeze for approximately 2 hours.

4. When frozen, twist your silicone molds and pop out your chips onto a small plate.

5. Serve!

Nutritional Value:

27.5 Calories.

0.2 grams of Protein.

0.1 grams of Carbs.

2.8 grams of Fat.

Homemade Nutella (Serves 12)

Ingredients:

2 cups of Hazelnuts

1/4 cup of Water

1 tablespoon of Coconut Oil

1/4 cup of Heavy Cream

1/4 cup of Cocoa Powder

1/2 cup of Erythritol

1 teaspoon of Vanilla Extract

1/4 teaspoon of Salt

Directions:

1. Preheat your oven to 325 degrees.

2. Spread your cookie sheet and spread your hazelnuts evenly in one layer. Roast for approximately 10 to 15 minutes.

3. Allow your nuts to cool. Put your nuts in a towel and rub them vigorously.

4. Once your nuts have their skins off, drop them into your food processor. Blend for a few minutes until it looks like peanut butter.

5. If sticking to sides add a little coconut oil and scrape down the sides.

6. Add in the rest of your ingredients. Continue to blend and scrape the sides.

7. Remove from your blender once thoroughly mixed and place in your container.

8. Serve!

Nutritional Value:

162 Calories.

3 grams of Protein.

2 grams of Carbs.

15 grams of Fat.

Nutella Brownies (Serves 4)

Ingredients:

4 Eggs

4 tablespoons of Erythritol

1 cup of Nutella

Directions:

1. Preheat your oven to 350 degrees.

2. Place your Nutella in your microwave for approximately 15-second intervals, stirring until it gets really soft.

3. Crack your eggs and mix with your electric mixer until they've tripled in volume and become a lighter yellow color. Should take approximately 5 to 8 minutes.

4. Combine your Nutella and eggs. Whisk until it is combined. Add your erythritol.

5. Add your mixture to ramekins. Put your ramekins on a cookie sheet. Bake approximately 25 to 30 minutes.

6. Allow it to cool.

7. Serve!

Nutritional Value:

396 Calories.

12 grams of Protein.

4 grams of Carbs.

35 grams of Fat.

Conclusion

Thanks for reading my book. I hope this recipe guide has provided you with all the recipes you needed to get going. Don't wait getting started. The sooner you start the sooner you'll begin to see an improvement in your health and well-being. While you won't see results overnight, they will start to come if you stick to the recipes found in this book.

There are so many options you can enjoy while on a ketogenic diet. I've tried to add a good mixture of recipes around each meal of the day including snacks and desserts. This way you'll have some healthy choices no matter what meal you're cooking for.

Best of luck. I wish you nothing but good fortune going forward!

21124295R00209

Printed in Great Britain
by Amazon